AMERICAN MEDICAL ASSOCIATION ESSENTIAL GUIDE TO
DEPRESSION

So often dismissed as a personality weakness or "all in one's head," depression is a serious illness that can disrupt the life of the depressed person and his or her family and friends, and take a physical and emotional toll. But it doesn't have to be that way; today, treatments for depression—and our understanding of its causes—are on the cutting edge of medical knowledge.

The American Medical Association brings its wealth of experience and scholarship to this down-to-earth, comprehensive reference. The guide begins with an illuminating overview of depression, supplemented by case studies, and a discussion of symptoms that may require medical attention. All forms of depressive illness and mood disorders are discussed in a detailed but accessible chapter. The most up-to-date information on the causes and contributing factors of depression is explained thoroughly, and the connection between depression and physical illnesses is fully explored.

Finally, the treatments for managing and overcoming all types of depression are presented in a clear, intelligible way. For anyone who is not sure where to turn for help, or those wishing to help a friend or loved one, the *American Medical Association Essential Guide to Depression* provides solid medical answers and manageable guidelines for seeking treatment.

American
Medical
Association

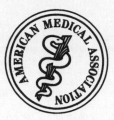

ESSENTIAL
GUIDE
TO
DEPRESSION

POCKET BOOKS
New York   London   Toronto   Sydney   Singapore

The information, procedures, and recommendations in this book are not intended as a substitute for the medical advice of a trained health professional. All matters regarding your health require medical supervision. Consult your physician before adopting the suggestions in this book, as well as about any condition that may require diagnosis or medical attention.

In addition, statements made by the author regarding certain products do not constitute an endorsement of any product, service, or organization by the author or publisher, each of whom specifically disclaims any responsibility for any liability, loss, or risk, personal or otherwise, which is incurred as a consequence, directly or indirectly, of the use and application of any of the contents of this book or any of the products mentioned herein.

An *Original* Publication of POCKET BOOKS

POCKET BOOKS, a division of Simon & Schuster Inc.
1230 Avenue of the Americas, New York, NY 10020

Library of Congress Cataloging-in-Publication Data

Essential guide to depression / American Medical Association.
   p. cm.
  Includes bibliographical references and index.
  ISBN: 0-671-01016-6
  1. Depression, Mental—Popular works. 2. Manic-depressive
illness—Popular works. 3. Consumer education. I. American
Medical Association.
RC537.E77   1998
616.85′27—dc21   98-19507
                                  CIP

First Pocket Books trade paperback printing September 1998

10 9 8 7 6 5 4 3

POCKET and colophon are registered trademarks of
Simon & Schuster Inc.

Cover design and cover photo by Elizabeth Van Itallie
Text design by Stanley S. Drate/Folio Graphics Co. Inc.

Printed in the U.S.A.

American Medical Association

Physicians dedicated to the health of America

Foreword

Undiagnosed and untreated depression is a major health problem today. Often it is difficult for people who have depression to admit that they have it and they need help. Or they may think they are simply feeling sad or have "the blues" temporarily, when in fact they have depression and could greatly benefit from treatment. Today's treatments include a variety of medications, along with psychotherapy and other "talking therapies." The *American Medical Association Essential Guide to Depression* is being published to make available medically accurate, clear, and up-to-date information on all facets of this disorder and its treatment.

As a potential reader for this volume, you may be wondering whether you have depression or if you are ready to seek treatment. Or, perhaps more commonly, you may be a family member or friend of someone who has depression; this volume accordingly contains helpful suggestions on how to convince that person to acknowledge the depression and get some help.

This book explains various types of depression, including major clinical depression, bipolar depression, seasonal affective disorder, and dysthymia. Also included are discussions of the various risk groups that are perhaps more likely to develop depression, or to be diagnosed for it, including older people, women, and teenagers. Also included are suggestions on how to recognize if someone is suicidal and how to help prevent suicide.

AMA member physicians offer this information to individuals and families struggling to overcome depression. If you have access to the Internet, look for more information about family health and about doctors on the AMA website at **http://www.ama-assn. org**; if you need a physician, you can access information by the doctor's name or by specialty under Physician Select: Online Doctor Finder.

We wish you and your family the best of mental health and physical health.

Nancy W. Dickey, MD
President, American Medical Association

The American Medical Association

Lynn E. Jensen, PhD, Chief Operating Officer
Robert L. Kennett, Senior Vice President,
  Publishing and Business Services
M. Frances Dyra, Director, Product Line Development

Editorial Staff

Angela Perry, MD, Medical Editor
Margaret Rukstalis, MD, Psychiatry
Patricia Dragisic, Managing Editor
Mark Ingebretsen, Senior Editor
Mary Feely, Writer
Barbara Scotese, Editor
Laura M. Barnes, Editorial Assistant

Acknowledgments

Patricia Ohlenroth
Linda Bresolin, PhD, American Medical Association
Janis Donnaud, Literary Agent
Larry Goldman, MD, American Medical Association

Contents

Contents

American
Medical
Association

ESSENTIAL
GUIDE
TO
DEPRESSION

Introduction

Depression is a serious illness, affecting about 17 million Americans each year, causing great pain not only to those who have depression but to their families and friends as well.

The good news is that like most illnesses, depression is treatable. However, many depressed people (nearly two thirds) do not recognize their illness and thus never receive the treatment they need. And many people do see depression not as an illness but as a weakness or flaw in their personalities.

In the *American Medical Association Essential Guide to Depression*, we present a comprehensive picture of depression, its causes, and its treatments. If you are depressed, we hope this book will encourage you to seek help. If you have a friend or a loved one who is depressed, we hope this book will provide you with strategies and information that you can use to help that person.

This book begins with a basic introduction to depression, complete with simulated case studies and facts and figures about depression. A chapter on types of depressive illness goes into the subject in more detail, defining the categories and types of depression and listing common symptoms.

People with depression and their families need and want information on what is known about why depression happens. The role that brain chemistry and hormones play is thoroughly explored, as is the contribution of genetic inheritance. Another important topic the book examines is depression that occurs at the same time as a physical illness.

This book explains how to find help for depression and what you may experience when you do. The book presents a wealth of detailed information on current treatments available, including medication and other therapies. A special chapter is devoted to helping a loved one who has depression. At the back of the book is a glossary of medical terms used, along with a list of mental health–related organizations and associations, many of which make information available to the consumer.

The *American Medical Association Guide to Depression* presents the information you need to help yourself or others. It is not always easy to begin treatment, but once you take the first steps, you and the people you care about will be on the road to recovery and good mental health.

1

Depression Defined

Theresa's eyes filled with tears. Ever since she had been promoted at work, it seemed that she was too tired to think. She felt so out of her depth in the new position that a fear of being demoted by her boss gripped her daily. She felt that if she lost this job, she would never get another one this good.

In the evenings, she dragged herself home. Her husband, Jeff, had gotten into the habit of making dinner just for himself because Theresa never seemed to be hungry. Her lack of appetite was making her lose weight these days. At one time, her weight loss would have made her proud, but not now. Lately, she had no interest in anything. She used to enjoy her sexual relationship with Jeff, but not now. She was too tired. Yet no matter how tired she was, she still woke up around 3 A.M. every day and thought about her failures. She could not remember when she had last felt happy. And she was beginning to wonder if anything good would ever happen to her again.

ED: GROUCHY AND ACHY

Ed poured his nightly glass of wine. He had never been much of a drinker when his wife was alive, but he needed a glass to make himself sleep at night. While he drank, he watched television just to hear the sound of another voice. He did not think of himself as lonely, though. His life was not great, but it was not bad either. It was just ordinary.

If he wanted to talk to somebody, he could always call his son, Steve. Steve seemed worried about him now that he was living alone. He should be grateful for Steve's concern, but instead, he felt annoyed. There was something very irritating about Steve's constant questions and invitations to come over for dinner and suggestions that he join a senior citizens' club. In fact, just about everyone got on Ed's nerves more than they used to. It was easier to be alone.

Ed winced at the familiar pain in his stomach. Maybe the nightly wine was doing damage. His back had been bothering him a lot, too, but that was to be expected at his age. Maybe the stomachache was just another part of getting old.

MICHELLE: HAPPY, HAPPY, HAPPY

This was the best time of Michelle's life in every way. She had always wanted to write a novel, and now she was finally doing it. The ideas flowed into her mind so quickly that it was hard to get them all down on paper. She felt inspired; she knew her novel was brilliant. And now she had ideas for a screenplay, too. Finally, after all these years, she was realizing her creative potential.

Her sense of joy spilled into every area of her life. Nothing could put her in a bad mood. She had always been a little shy, but now she found it easy to approach strangers and start a conversation. The other day, she had overheard two neighbors talking about home repairs, and she had happily joined in. She had ended up doing most of the talking. She was more assertive sexually these days, too. She enjoyed letting men know she found them attractive.

Michelle had more energy than ever, no matter how hard she worked. After a couple of hours of sleep, she awoke completely refreshed. Michelle felt that she could accomplish anything. For once, she was so certain of success that she was willing to buy anything she wanted, no matter what the cost. She just charged it, whether she could afford it or not. She deserved good things. Nothing was beyond her.

Theresa, Ed, and Michelle are all behaving very differently, but they all have one thing in common. Theresa's unrelenting sadness and exhaustion, Ed's stomachache and irritability, and even Michelle's endless buoyancy and energy are all signs of one of the most common and destructive disorders in the US— depression.

WHAT IS DEPRESSION?

Depression is a type of mental disorder that disturbs a person's mood. Human moods can be thought of as a kind of rainbow: each mood is distinct, yet each one blends into the next. The shades of this rainbow range from severe depression through mild depression, normal sadness, everyday moods, mild mania, and mania (euphoria mixed with behavior problems). Everyone moves through various shades of the rainbow; it is normal and appropriate to respond to such events as the loss of a job or a loved one with sad, gloomy feelings. When these feelings become inappropriate, extreme, and dysfunctional, however, they are seen as a mood disorder.

Because depression often goes untreated, doctors are not sure exactly how many people have the illness. They know, however, that it is far from rare. In fact, depression is so widespread that it is sometimes called the "common cold of mental illness."

The term *depression* is often used to describe feelings of deep sadness. Almost everyone experiences sadness at one time or another. But people with depressive illness—sometimes called major depression, major depressive disorder, or clinical depression to distinguish it from ordinary sadness—experience an overwhelming and debilitating despondency that is long lasting and typically interferes with a person's life at home, in the workplace, or in social situations. When healthy people feel dejected by everyday events—a fight with a loved one, a rejection for a job promotion, a move from a familiar home—they may say, "I feel depressed." But the feeling they call "depression" is distinct from the clinical disease of depression. Normal sadness, no matter how painful, usually goes away over time without special treatment. People who are sad can live their everyday lives despite their sorrow. By contrast, depressive illness does not fade so easily and can seriously interrupt a person's ability to think and act.

Left untreated, major depression can be dangerous. Suicidal thoughts are a common part of this illness. Although deeply depressed people rarely have the energy to commit suicide, they may be more likely to do so as their depression begins to subside. Untreated depression is the most common cause of suicide in the US.

In some people, periods of depression alternate with periods of extreme joy and dysfunctional behavior known as mania. Such people have a kind of depressive illness called bipolar disorder or manic depression, or manic-depressive illness. This illness can make you hyperactive, irritable, and excessively self-confident. In addition, it can destroy your normal judgment and cause reckless behavior. Michelle's feelings of invincibility and wild spending habits, for example, are all symptoms of her mania.

Cyclothymia, also called cyclothymic disorder, is a milder but more lasting form of bipolar depression. People with cyclothymia have moods that swing between hypomania (a mild form of mania) and mild depression.

Like major depression, bipolar depression can be dangerous. During the depressed phase of your illness, you may be haunted by thoughts of suicide. During the manic phase of your illness, your good judgment may evaporate and you may not be able to see the harm of your actions. You may incur huge credit card debts, for example, or become sexually promiscuous. In some cases, people with mania lose touch with reality.

Milder, less common forms of depression include dysthymia, also called dysthymic disorder or depressive neurosis, and minor depression, also called minor depressive disorder. Recurrent brief depressive disorder feels like major depression but lasts for only a brief time. Postpartum depression is a depressive illness that develops in new mothers about 1 week to 6 months after the birth of their babies. Premenstrual dysphoric disorder is a cyclic illness that affects 3 percent to 5 percent of menstruating women. Women with this illness feel extremely depressed and irritable for a week or two before menstruation each month. Seasonal affective disorder (SAD) is a type of depression that occurs only at certain times of the year. People with this illness typically feel lethargic and depressed during winter months, yet their moods are normal during the summer months. Atypical depression has a mix of depressive symptoms that do not fit in perfectly with any of the existing categories.

In all its guises, depression distorts the way people view themselves, others, and the world. Theresa's thoughts are warped by self-loathing. Ed's irritability is damaging his relationships with other people. While Michelle's illness may seem to have positive aspects, it is clouding her judgment and making her act recklessly. In each of these cases, depressive illness is preventing people from leading their everyday lives.

No matter how their symptoms may vary, people with depressive illness find it affects almost every aspect of their lives, from how well they concentrate at work to how deeply they sleep at night. Eventually, it can make ordinary life impossible. But depression, in all its forms, can be treated. Major depression is one of the most treatable illnesses. Bipolar depression has no cure but can be controlled with medication. Other types of depression are also treatable.

The different types of depressive illness are discussed more fully in Chapter 2. Treatments are discussed in Chapters 5 and 6.

Am I Depressed or Just Blue?

If you are coping with a major loss, such as the death of your spouse or partner, you will experience some symptoms of depression. For example, you may find it hard to fall asleep, you may have no appetite for food, and you may have difficulty concentrating during the day. During a period of mourning after a major loss, such symptoms of depression are normal. Chances are you are enduring normal grief which, though difficult, is healthy.

Normal grief tends to go through stages, during which you react to your loss by first denying it, then coming to terms with it, and eventually accepting it. Immediately after the death of a loved one, for example, you may react with tears or pretend that he or she is still alive. You make funeral arrangements but your actions feel unreal, as if you were watching a movie. You cannot believe this has happened to you. You may feel completely numb.

Later, these feelings change as you acknowledge the reality of your loss. This is when you may experience sleeplessness, fatigue, lack of appetite, or other symptoms of depression. You may also feel guilty, disorganized, bewildered, and despairing. Activities you used to enjoy have no appeal. You may avoid family and friends. The memory of your loved one may preoccupy you, and you may yearn to see him or her just one more time. Perhaps you fantasize about dying and joining your loved one. (Thoughts of suicide are *not* usually part of the normal grieving process; see "Do I Need Help?"[pages 116 through 119] in Chapter 5, "Getting Help for Depression.") Slowly, however, your feelings change as you come to accept your loss. You still miss the person who died, but you regain your interest in other people. You care about whether your clothes are clean or your hair is tidy. A tasty meal or a sunny day gives you pleasure again.

At some point during your mourning, your grief can begin to make a great impact on your life. Sometimes, normal grief motivates people to change their lives. If your loved one was murdered, for example, you might become active in a group that lobbies for changes in the sentencing of convicted murderers. You might start to devote much of your spare time to the work or favorite charity of the person who died, or even make your loved one's work your full-time occupation.

Other people may react to a loss, particularly a loss of health or mobility after a serious illness, by becoming demoralized. People in this situation can experience some symptoms of depression, including low self-esteem, feelings of hopelessness, or a heightened sense that life is out of control. People with cancer, heart disease, or serious burns often experience such loss of spirit. The person's spirit generally returns when self-esteem improves during rehabilitation therapy.

Of course, many of us who have not endured a great loss still feel blue from time to time. Perhaps you lost your car keys on Monday, were denied a pay raise on Tuesday, and had to cope with blocked drains on Wednesday. Now you feel as if nothing will ever go right. Or maybe you have just returned to a difficult job after a delightful vacation and you now think that you have absolutely nothing to look forward to. You may feel pessimistic and grouchy for no very good reason. These moods are normal, provided you can continue to lead your life.

If you feel low in spirit but continue to do your work well and maintain your relationships with family and friends, you are not clinically depressed. Sadness and anxiety are often healthy reactions to losses, large or small. For at least 2 months after your loss, these symptoms are considered normal. But healthy grief that persists and remains severe for a long time after a loss can slowly deepen into clinical depression. If you are clinically depressed, you will not function normally. Your symptoms will be longer lasting, more extreme, and less likely to improve without treatment, and they will prevent you from behaving normally at work or in social situations.

An important difference between normal sadness and clinical depression is the effect your condition has on your self-esteem. People with clinical depression contend with constant negative thoughts about themselves, their lives, and their futures. Hopelessness paralyzes them. They may think that nothing ever works for them, that nothing ever will. They feel stuck, unable to act, and unable to relate to other people. People experiencing normal sadness or a negative mood may brood about their situation, but basically they are the people they have always been. Despite everything, they feel active and alive.

For example, a healthy person just fired from a job may think, "I feel terrible about losing that job. The money was good and I liked the work. Plus, I was good at it. I did not deserve to be fired." A clinically depressed person, by contrast, may think, "How can I survive without my job? I know I will never get another. I am a terrible person and a total loser." The healthy person's outlook is an honest and realistic assessment of the situation, while the depressed person's outlook is overly negative and unrealistic and may lead to an inability to take action.

FACTS AND FIGURES ABOUT DEPRESSION

Research has shown that in a given year, at least 17.5 million American adults—1 in 10—will experience depression and that there is a depressed person in an estimated 1 in 5 families.

Some forms of depression are more common than others. Major depression is likely to affect about 15 percent of Americans at least once in their lifetimes. Bipolar disorder is thought to occur in at least 1.2 percent of the population, or more than 3 million people. Milder versions of these illnesses may affect a further 2 percent to 5 percent of Americans. Particular groups of people are also more likely than others to develop depressive illness. Women, for example, experience depression at roughly twice the rate that men do. Depression is found in all age groups but occurs most frequently in middle-aged adults.

Depressive illness may be growing more prevalent in the US. Research shows that more people are now developing depression at an earlier age. For example, of the generation born between 1940 and 1959, about 10 percent may have experienced an episode of depression by the age of 25. Of the generation born before 1940, only 2.5 percent experienced depression by age 25. Researchers are uncertain how to interpret these statistics. Doctors may be better at diagnosing depression in young people today than they were in the past, or older people may not accurately remember when they first experienced depression.

Depression is costly, in both economic and human terms. The economic cost of depression ranges from $15 billion to $35 billion a year in lost time and productivity, employee turnover, and medical care. We have no way to measure its human cost. Untreated, the disease damages self-esteem, promotes substance abuse, disrupts relationships and careers, and sometimes causes disability or even death.

Many depressed people today fail to recognize depression in themselves. Indeed, certain symptoms of depression may even prevent a person from seeking help. If you experience the feelings of self-loathing common in depression, you may blame yourself for your low feelings. If you experience fatigue also, which is common, seeing a doctor may seem too exhausting to attempt. If you feel the unwarranted invincibility of mania, you may reject even the possibility of illness.

But even among those who recognize their illness, many decline to get help. Doctors estimate that two thirds of people who have depression fail to seek treatment. The reasons for this vary, but many people do not seek treatment simply because the illness is misunderstood. It may be seen as a sign of weakness. However, depressive illness is no more a personal failing than is heart disease, high blood pressure, or any other medical condition. It cannot be shaken off at will. Sometimes when people have the blues over some temporary setback or disappointment, it helps for them to keep busy or make an effort to pull out of their momentary feeling. But this is not true for depression. Without medical care, depression can last for weeks, months, or years.

Yet depression is a highly treatable illness. Doctors can remove or reduce all the symptoms of depression in more than 80 percent of their patients. But the longer the illness goes undetected and untreated, the more difficult it becomes to treat. Severe, untreated depression can result in suicide. People whose depression is severe enough to require hospitalization have a suicide rate as high as 15 percent.

Such statistics may seem daunting. But doctors today know far more about depression—its possible causes and effective treatments—than they knew even 20 years ago.

WHO IS AT RISK FOR DEPRESSION?

To some extent, we all run the risk of depressive illness. Depression has been diagnosed in all kinds of people: rich and poor, young and old, married and single. Stressful events come along in every life, and if these events are sufficiently severe and numerous, they may trigger depressive illness. We are also all vulnerable to physical ailments and have the potential to develop a disorder that later gives rise to depression. While no one is entirely immune to depressive illness, the most common forms—major depression and bipolar depression—do affect some groups of people more than others.

Gender Factors

Women are diagnosed and treated for major depression more often than men. In the US, a woman is about twice as likely as a man to be diagnosed with depression. Researchers have found that depression is equally common among male and female children, but during adolescence, girls start to show more depression than boys. This vulnerability continues throughout a woman's adult life. Even in old age, more women than men have depressive illness. In the US, about 20 percent to 25 percent of women will become seriously depressed at least once in their lives. Of men, about 12 percent will do so.

Doctors do not fully understand why they treat more depressed women than men, but they have several theories. One is that women are more prone to depression because they have more stress than do men. Women today have to cope with conflicting roles, with demanding schedules at work and at home. Some experts believe the traits encouraged in girls as they grow up, such as a willingness to please others rather than themselves, may later make them prone to depression.

Another explanation is that it is not that depression is actually more widespread among women but that women are more likely to seek treatment. Women may be willing to acknowledge the emotional symptoms of depression, such as feeling sad, lonely, or hopeless. According to this theory, men are less inclined to admit to such feelings. Also, doctors who diagnose depression may be biased and more likely to look for it in women than in men. Some researchers suspect that such a bias may account for the fact that women make up about 60 percent of medical patients yet receive about 75 percent of all prescriptions for mood-altering drugs.

Some theories suggest that men may try to stifle their depression with alcohol or other substances instead of seeking medical help. The depression may be masked—that is, seen as the result of the alcohol or drug dependency rather than as a separate disorder. As a result, men may be less likely to be treated for depression.

The idea that depressive illness is overlooked in men is supported by research on depression among Amish people in Pennsylvania. The Amish people are members of a Protestant religion that requires personal simplicity and withdrawal from the modern world. Amish farming communities typically are self-reliant and tightly knit, and large families and cooperation among neighbors are common. Studies have shown that depression is equally common among Amish men and women. One possible explanation of this is that Amish men cannot mask their depression with drugs or alcohol because such substances are strictly forbidden by their religion. Also, the close ties among Amish people may ensure that any unusual behavior is promptly noted and treated.

Another theory is that women are more vulnerable to depression because their bodies experience a constant ebb and flow of hormones. Hormones are chemicals produced by certain organs and glands in the body that control many of the body's processes, including growth, metabolism, and sexual development. Hormonal levels shift routinely during a woman's monthly menstrual cycle. In some women, there may be a link between depression and these cyclic changes. Times of particularly great hormonal change in women include pregnancy, the time immediately after giving birth, and menopause, the period of a woman's life when her menstrual cycles become increasingly infrequent and then stop. For a few women, some of these milestones are marked by depressive illness.

Studies disagree over the relationship between pregnancy and depression. It appears, however, that pregnant women who are especially prone to depression are those who have unhappy marriages, who do not want a baby, and who have a history of depression or relatives with depression. Many women experience short-lived "blues" in the first few days after giving birth. Few women go on to develop full-blown depressive illness during the period after childbirth.

Menopause was once thought to be a time of depression. In fact, doctors regarded such depression as a unique disorder that they called involutional melancholia. Today, we know that it is not a unique disorder and that in general, women do not always develop it during menopause. Women who do develop it at that time typically have had a history of depressive illness.

Among women, rates of major depression are highest among the unhappily married, separated, and divorced, and lowest among the happily married. And though depression is cross-cultural, it appears that doctors in the US diagnose depression less frequently in African American women than in white women and more frequently in Hispanic women. One possible explanation of this, researchers believe, is that African American women are more likely to complain of the physical symptoms of depression than of the mood changes that go with it. This may be based on cultural issues about seeking out psychiatric help.

In contrast to major depression, bipolar disorder affects men and women equally. Why depression is found overwhelmingly in women, while mania is not, is unclear. But it may be that mania is simply more likely to be noticed than depression because of its striking symptoms. Also, it could be that depression is simply overlooked in men.

Creativity as a Risk Factor

Artists and writers, as a group are more likely to experience depression than other groups. Artists believed to have had depressive illness include writers Ernest Hemingway, Leo Tolstoy, and William Styron; poets Sylvia Plath, Anne Sexton, and Walt Whitman; and painters Georgia O'Keeffe, Vincent Van Gogh, and Jackson Pollock. Some scientific studies claim to confirm a link between artistic achievement and depressive illness. For example, one study compared 30 members of the University of Iowa Writers' Workshop with a group of nonwriters. Depressive illness was far more common among the writers—about 80 percent had either depression or mania, compared with 30 percent of the nonwriters. A separate study of leading British writers found that more than one third of the participants had been treated for depressive illness. These studies are far from conclusive, however, and much research must be done to confirm any link between depression and creativity.

If creativity and depressive illness are in fact linked, the exact connection between the two is unclear. It is less likely that creative work will be produced while an artist is experiencing depression, mania, or hypomania. Researchers found that many artists were unable to work while depressed and that artists produced poor work during mania. In addition, the artists found it hard to concentrate and were easily distracted during hypomania.

Age Factors

Depression and mania can affect people at any age, but symptoms are more likely to appear for the first time at certain stages of life. For example, you are most likely to experience your first episode of mania while in your teens or twenties. Depression also generally emerges for the first time in adults. In about half of depressed people, the illness first occurs between the ages of 20 and 50.

Although depression typically emerges for the first time in

young people, older people as a group seem particularly susceptible. Estimates of how many older people have depressive illness vary widely. According to one estimate, about 15 percent of people over 65 years of age have some symptoms. Their symptoms may be mistakenly interpreted as due to physical problems instead of depression. People living in nursing homes seem to be especially at risk.

There are many possible reasons for this high rate of depression among older people. Older people typically have gone through a number of losses, such as diminished health, the death of a spouse or partner or friends, or lowered income after retirement. In addition, depression can be part of physical illnesses that are more common in this age group, such as cardiovascular disease. Also, depression is sometimes a side effect of prescription drugs, which are used more frequently by older people—those over 65 take an average of seven or more medications each day. Depression may be a side effect of one such medication or a combination of several medications.

Other Factors

Your chances of getting depression or mania increase if you have had the illness before. Estimates vary, but about half of people who have depression once develop the illness again. In bipolar disorder, most people who have had one episode will experience a second.

You are also more likely to develop depressive illness if you have a relative who has had a depressive illness. This is especially true of bipolar depression. According to some scientific studies, immediate family members—parents, siblings, or children—of people with bipolar depression are 8 to 18 times more likely than the close relatives of healthy people to develop the illness. In addition, having a close family member with bipolar depression may make you more vulnerable to major depression. According to some studies, immediate family members of people with bipolar depression are 2 to 10 times more likely to have major depression than are the close relatives of healthy people. Likewise, if you have a close relative with major depression, you may be twice as likely to develop bipolar or major depression than other people.

Your ethnic background does not seem to affect your chances of developing depression or mania. It may affect your chances of receiving the proper diagnosis and treatment, however. Studies have shown that doctors are less likely to recognize mood disorders in people from an ethnic group that is different culturally from their own. A doctor of a particular ethnic group may perceive behavior that is accepted among people of another ethnic group as eccentric or abnormal.

In men and women, depressive illness is more common in people who are divorced, separated, or have no close relationships. Depressive illness puts great strain on relationships, and people who are alone often lack an emotional support system. Also, bipolar depression usually first emerges in youth, and people with this illness may have fewer opportunities to date or get married. Depression also seems to be common in widows and widowers. One study, for example, found signs of depression in about one sixth of widows and widowers 1 year after the death of a spouse or partner.

Certain personality traits may make you more vulnerable to depression. If you tend to criticize yourself, take a pessimistic approach toward life, or depend unduly on other people, you may be more prone to depression than happy-go-lucky types. A person who is withdrawn and reluctant to reach out to other people may also be at risk. By themselves, these traits certainly do not cause depression. But suppose, for example, you have a genetic predisposition to depression and have recently experienced several losses. Your inability to reach out to other people in this situation may put you at a higher risk for depression than a person who can easily ask for help.

Certain losses may make depression more likely later in life. The loss of a parent or significant loved one before the age of 11 may make you more prone to depression as an adult. People who have gone through other catastrophic losses, survived disasters, or participated in combat during a war are also at risk. Losses and other painful experiences themselves probably do not cause the depression, but they may result in a lifelong vulnerability or accentuate a genetic vulnerability.

Depression and mania can affect people in all social classes. Depression appears to be equally common among the rich and the poor. Bipolar disorder is most often diagnosed in people of comfortable means, perhaps because they have greater access to health care. Bipolar disorder is also more common among those without a college degree than among college graduates. This may be because the illness typically develops at an early age and is likely to interfere with a person's studies.

Although some people seem more prone to depressive illness than others do, no one is predestined to become ill. Many children of depressed people, for example, never develop the illness despite being at risk. Knowing that you are at risk for developing depressive illness may motivate you to learn more about the illness, to be alert for its warning signs, and to take steps to lessen your vulnerability—by avoiding excessive amounts of stress, for example. Far from making depression inevitable, knowing the risks can help you beat it.

2

Types of Depressive Illness

Like many medical conditions, depressive illness takes different forms. The most common are major depression and bipolar depression, but several less common forms also exist. Also, depression varies in degree. Mild depression occurs when you have some symptoms and must push yourself to carry out your day-to-day activities. Moderate depression exists when you have many symptoms and often cannot do the things you need to do. Severe depression is present when you have nearly all the symptoms and have serious difficulties in coping with ordinary, everyday life.

All types of depression belong to a group of illnesses known as mood disorders or major affective disorders. Each type has a distinct pattern of symptoms.

MAJOR DEPRESSION

Major depression—also known as major depressive disorder, unipolar depression, or clinical depression—is the most common type of depressive illness. The term *unipolar,* meaning one pole or extreme of emotion, is used to describe this illness because it is marked by a single mood of sadness. (Bipolar depression, discussed later in this chapter, has two poles or extremes of emotion, sadness and euphoria.)

Major depression affects different people in different ways. Most people with major depression feel persistently sad, lose pleasure in activities they used to enjoy, or experience a combination of the two. These emotional changes go hand in hand with such mental and physical changes as sleeplessness, forgetfulness or inability to concentrate, a loss of appetite, and aches and pains.

The feelings of major depression vary, but most people with the illness experience deep emotional pain. Major depression can make you feel worthless, hopeless, and helpless. It can weigh you down with guilt. Many people describe their feelings of depression as a black cloud or dark shadow over their lives.

No one knows exactly what causes major depression. Some people develop the illness after going through great hardships. Others fall ill when everything seems to be going well in their lives. One theory is that abnormal activity in the chemistry of the brain gives rise to the illness. In some people, a tendency to develop the disorder may be inherited. In others, depression may be linked to abnormal levels of hormones in the body. Still another cause of depression may be a mistimed biological clock. This term is commonly used for the body's timing mechanism that controls the rhythms of certain functions and processes in the body, such as a regular rise and fall of body temperature. Causes of depression are discussed more fully in Chapters 3 and 4.

Who Gets Major Depression?

Many people in the US have or have had major depression. Between 10 percent and 25 percent of us will be depressed at some point in our lives. Probably 5 percent to 6 percent of us are grappling with major depression right now. Major depression can affect anyone, at any age and in any circumstance, but in general, it first appears in people between the ages of 25 and 44. It is unusual to experience a first bout of depression after your late forties, although it becomes a little more likely as you move into your sixties because you typically face the major transitions of retirement and physical changes due to aging.

Characteristics of Major Depression

If you have major depression, you will not always feel depressed. Depression weighs you down for a certain length of time and then goes. Doctors call such periods of depression episodes. In most people, an episode of depression will lift within 6 to 9 months, even if it is not treated and no matter what caused it. You will probably feel your old self again once the depression leaves, although one of four people diagnosed with depression complains of lingering symptoms. Doctors do not fully understand the process through which depression eases without treatment. One theory is that the human body and mind have a natural tendency to correct abnormal conditions.

When depression is linked to an illness, a doctor may treat

the depression as an illness in its own right or may decide to first treat the medical condition that gave rise to it. For example, depression is a symptom of hypothyroidism. In this disorder, the thyroid gland fails to produce enough thyroid hormones, which regulate metabolism (the body's fuel-burning processes) and levels of calcium in the blood. Once the hypothyroidism clears, the depression is likely to clear as well. (See Chapter 4 for more information on secondary causes of depression.)

In some cases, major depression may be masked if it exists with a second disorder, such as alcoholism. A person who tries to alleviate his or her depression with alcohol may be seen as one who is depressed as a result of alcohol dependency, rather than the other way around. That person may receive treatment for alcoholism but may not fully recover unless the underlying disorder of depression is also treated (see Chapter 4).

An estimated one half of people who have one episode of major depression will experience a second. Depression that returns is called recurring or recurrent depression. In recurrent brief depressive disorder, the symptoms are as severe as in major depression, but they last for less than about 2 weeks.

Depression is more likely to return in some people than others, especially in people who have their first episode before their twenties and those for whom depression runs in the family. Your chance of depression's returning goes up with every episode. The more episodes you have, the more likely you are to have another.

Symptoms of Major Depression

No single diagnostic test can show that you have depressive illness, though some laboratory tests may help confirm a diagnosis of major depression. Instead, doctors look for a group of symptoms that together may point to depression. Depressive illness is a kind of medical condition known as a syndrome, meaning it is characterized by a collection of symptoms.

The signs of depression fall into four main categories: mood disturbances, such as overwhelming sadness or guilt; changes in behavior, such as withdrawal from other people; altered thinking, or cognition, such as lack of concentration; and physical complaints, such as insomnia. Physical signs of depression are sometimes called vegetative or somatic symptoms. Your symptoms of depression will vary with your age and other aspects of your life. If you are a middle-aged adult, for example, you may complain of unremitting sadness. Older people, however, are more likely to experience the physical symptoms of depressive illness. Children often reveal their depression through behavioral changes, such as losing interest in friends and school.

Because depressive illness affects your mood and thoughts, you may find it hard to accurately assess your symptoms. If you think you may be depressed, ask close friends or family members whether they have noticed changes in your mood, behavior, thinking, or physical health. They may have seen something that you are not aware of, such as frequent nervous gestures. Also, your symptoms will be worse at some times compared to others. Many depressed people feel terrible in early morning but gradually improve throughout the day. Others feel worse as the day wears on. Doctors refer to this daily ebb and flow of depression as a diurnal variation of mood. Some depressed women notice a worsening of symptoms in the days before their menstrual period begins.

The two main signs of depression are persistent feelings of

sadness and a loss of interest or pleasure in things you used to enjoy. You must have at least one of these symptoms for at least 2 weeks for depressive illness to be diagnosed. In addition, these moods must be severe enough to prevent you from functioning normally at work or in social situations. They must also occur with four or more other symptoms from the following list that you experience nearly every day:

- Significant weight loss when not dieting, significant weight gain, loss of appetite, or increased appetite
- Inability to sleep or oversleeping
- Physical movements that are more restless or slower than usual
- Fatigue or loss of energy
- Feelings of worthlessness or inappropriate guilt
- Inability to think clearly, concentrate, or make decisions
- Recurrent thoughts of death, ideas of suicide without a specific plan, a plan to commit suicide, or a suicide attempt

You may experience any combination of these symptoms during depression. If they sound familiar, talk to your doctor.

Often, the person fails to recognize that he or she has depression and may resist suggestions about depression from friends and family. If you are concerned that a family member needs help, talk to your doctor for suggestions on how to approach the person. See Chapter 5 for more information on getting help for depression for yourself, a family member, or a friend.

SADNESS

Most clinically depressed people feel blue, empty, hopeless, or worthless. Their bleak despondency is more acute than ordinary sadness—it is agonizing emotional pain. If you are depressed, you may think your life has been drained of everything good. You may be unable to remember happy times or imagine feeling joyful again. Despite your distress, you may be unable to cry. The ability to cry often returns as the depression improves. Other depressed people, however, may be tearful most of the day, especially in the early stages of depression. The dark mood that is characteristic of depression is sometimes called dysphoric mood or dysphoria. Another term for this overwhelming sadness and grief is melancholia.

Not all people with depressive illness describe sadness, however. Children and adolescents may reveal their depression through an irritable, rather than despondent, mood. Young people who are depressed may be cranky or bad tempered most of the time. Rather than saying they feel sad, they may say they feel ugly, stupid, or useless. Some depressed adults feel grouchy, hostile, or angry rather than sad. Older people are more likely to complain of physical aches and pains than a depressed mood.

Many depressed people withdraw emotionally from others. You may no longer enjoy eating lunch with coworkers or classmates. At home, you may sit silently through the family dinner and escape to bed as soon as possible. Chances are, you resent your loved one's attempts to discuss your behavior. The other symptoms you experience may foster this reduced social contact. For example, if you feel tired all the time, you will not feel much like joining friends for a shopping excursion. And if you are sad most of the day, you may avoid coworkers out of fear that you may become tearful in their presence.

LOSS OF PLEASURE

If you are depressed, you probably no longer enjoy any of the things that used to be fun. This lack of pleasure in normally pleasurable activities is sometimes called anhedonia. Your favorite television show, a fine wine, a walk on a spring day, an evening out with your closest friends—all leave you cold. Your work, in which you used to take satisfaction, may seem pointless. Some depressed people say the world seems drained of color.

During depression, your interest in sex may be diminished. Some people find a low sexual drive is the first warning sign of their illness. If you are depressed, sex may seem like far too much bother. You may be unable to remember what once made sex so enjoyable. Or you may attempt sexual intercourse but have difficulty achieving an erection or reaching orgasm. Other aspects of depression may also lessen your sexual appetite. For example, your low self-esteem may make you doubt that your spouse or partner is genuinely attracted to you.

CHANGES IN EATING HABITS

During depression, your attitude toward food usually changes. You may never feel hungry, even after going without food for several hours. One or two bites may be enough to fill you up. The thought of food may disgust you. Or, you may simply forget to eat. You may eat when somebody urges you to do so but without savoring or really tasting the food. Maybe you know you should be eating more, but the idea of buying and preparing food seems far too exhausting. One symptom of depression is losing 5 percent or more of your body weight in a single month while not following a reduced-calorie or reduced-fat diet. Depressed children may fail to make weight gains expected for their ages.

However, some depressed people find their appetite is greater than usual. You may find yourself eating more than ever, perhaps craving a certain type of food. People with seasonal affective disorder (SAD), for example, often crave such carbohydrates as bread, pasta, and potatoes. A sweet tooth can be part of bipolar disorder. Doctors sometimes refer to an increased appetite as an atypical feature of depression. A weight gain of 5 percent or more over your normal body weight in 1 month may also be a sign of depression.

These changes in appetite may bother you. They can cause harm in people who have a physical illness that requires a specific diet, such as diabetes or high blood pressure.

CHANGES IN SLEEPING HABITS

About 80 percent of depressed people also have trouble sleeping, which is called insomnia. The sleep problems of depression vary. It may take you longer than usual to fall asleep at night or you may be able to fall asleep but wake up several times at night. You may feel worried or anxious when you awaken, or you may lie awake for hours, brooding over your perceived failures. An especially common problem is waking early in the morning, perhaps as early as 3 A.M. The medical terms for this type of waking are *terminal insomnia* and *late-night insomnia*. Some people with depressive illness have learned that early awakening can be the first warning that their depression may be returning.

A small number of depressed people crave sleep. If you have SAD, for example, you may sleep longer during the winter. Even after 14 hours of sleep, you may feel sluggish and tired. The medical term for sleeping too much is *hypersomnia*.

PHYSICAL CHANGES

During depression, your physical movements may change. The most common change is slowing down. Your shoulders may slump as you sit. You may avert your eyes from other people, preferring to look at the ground. When you do move, it may be more slowly than usual. You may speak extremely slowly and use fewer words. When somebody talks to you, you make take 2 or 3 minutes to answer with a single word. Doctors call this slowing down of your movements psychomotor retardation.

By contrast, some people with depression find it impossible to sit still. Some walk up and down a room, again and again. Others develop nervous gestures, such as constantly cracking their knuckles or pulling their hair. Doctors refer to these speeded-up movements as psychomotor agitation. Older people are more likely to develop restless gestures than are younger people. Changes in physical movements may point toward depression, but they must be obvious to other people. Thus, if you feel slower than usual but your movements look normal to your doctor, you do not have this symptom of depression.

Almost all people with depression complain of reduced energy. You may feel tired all the time. Such routine tasks as emptying the dishwasher or writing a letter may seem exhausting. Starting a new project, whether it is painting the kitchen or changing the oil in your car, may seem utterly impossible. As a result of this feeling of lethargy, many people with depression find their work at home, office, or school suffers.

Many depressed people have chronic aches and pains, especially headaches, stomachaches, and back pain. Others are prone to gastrointestinal complaints, such as constipation, indigestion, and irritable bowel syndrome. Women with depression may experience painful or irregular menstrual periods. Some depressed people seek medical help for these physical problems rather than for the underlying depression. About 50 percent of depressed people complain to their doctors of physical ailments without mentioning mood changes. If you have chronic aches and pains, you may have depression even if you are unaware of extreme sadness. Doctors call this illness masked depression. With masked depression, the pain you feel is real, but it is caused by your state of mind rather than a physical illness.

DISTORTED EMOTIONS AND THOUGHTS

Depression has a powerful effect upon your thoughts and emotions. If you are depressed, your thoughts are likely to be very negative. You may feel unable to help yourself and certain that you will never feel well again.

If you are depressed, you probably no longer think the way you used to. Your thoughts may be confused or slower than usual. You may find it hard to focus on a particular task. A simple decision like choosing which shirt to wear may be very difficult. Perhaps you have become forgetful. You may be the only one who notices these changes, or they may be clear to others also.

Anxiety affects up to 90 percent of depressed people. With anxiety, some unnamed fear may overwhelm you. Worries, real and imagined, may occupy your thoughts. Perhaps you routinely expect something bad to happen. If your phone rings, for example, you may expect to hear bad news.

People with depression have thoughts and emotions that are distorted; that is, they do not reflect reality. In severe cases, these distorted thoughts may develop into delusions. A delusion is a firm belief in something despite factual evidence to the contrary. Doctors classify such delusions into two groups. One type of delusion is sad in tone or content. Another type is happy in tone or content. With the first type of delusion, a depressed woman might think she is extremely impoverished even if she is financially comfortable. With the second type, a depressed man might believe he is a powerful religious leader. In rare cases, people with depression may experience hallucinations—that is, seeing, hearing, feeling, tasting, or smelling something that is not there.

People with depression may also have low self-esteem or strong feelings of worthlessness or guilt. These feelings are distinct from a normal reaction of sadness. Say that you develop a chronic illness and can no longer work full time. Some feelings of sadness and regret may be appropriate. Excessive guilt, however, may develop into an illusion. For example, if you are deeply depressed, you may become convinced that God is punishing you by making you ill and that this punishment is deserved in some way.

The self-loathing common in depression may be fed by other symptoms. For example, you may feel too exhausted to open your mail and routinely toss your bills aside without paying them. Later, when creditors call to demand payment, you may turn this embarrassment inward and berate yourself for being a deadbeat. In addition, this symptom may make you less likely to seek medical help. You may see all the changes in yourself, from your constant exhaustion to your lack of enthusiasm for your daughter's cheerleading routine, as proof that you are an unworthy person. In fact, they are signs that you are ill.

Because depression distorts your thinking, making you see the bad over the good, it may also affect your attitude toward medical help. For example, you may think your symptoms are more severe than they are, and you may dismiss the idea that they can be treated.

Such mistaken thinking may lead you to misinform your doctor. For example, you may tell your doctor that a certain treatment was ineffective during a previous episode of depression, even if it was quite helpful. In your depressed state, you honestly remember the experience as negative. For this reason, your doctor may try to confirm any information you provide with a third person.

Depressed people are often preoccupied with death. About two thirds of depressed people think about suicide. Some are unable to think of anything else. Between 10 percent and 15 percent of people being treated for major depression eventually commit suicide. Those who are severely depressed generally lack the energy and motivation to kill themselves. However, they are more at risk as their depression begins to subside and their energy increases. People who wish they were dead but have a reason for living, such as the desire to raise their small children, may be less likely to commit suicide. At high risk are those who definitely plan to kill themselves and whose mood lightens after making that decision. People in this state of mind usually need to be hospitalized for their own safety.

Thoughts about suicide may lead to action. If you have thoughts about killing yourself, whether a detailed plan or a simple wish that you were dead, let your doctor and your family know.

Treatment of Major Depression

Treatment for major depression is widely available. It includes medication; psychotherapy with a psychotherapist, psychologist, psychoanalyst, or counselor; or a combination of treatments. Which treatment you choose will depend on the severity of your symptoms and your preference. Some doctors say that psychotherapy is as effective as medication in helping people with mild to moderate depression. If your depression is more severe, your doctor is likely to recommend a combination of medication and psychotherapy. Medication can relieve your physical symptoms quickly, while psychotherapy may teach you new ways to think about your life. Treatments are discussed in depth in Chapters 5 and 6.

VARIATIONS OF MAJOR DEPRESSION

There are several less common forms of major depression, called subtypes. They include psychotic depression, atypical depression, postpartum depression, postpartum psychosis, and premenstrual dysphoric disorder.

Psychotic Depression

People with psychotic depression have delusions or hallucinations in addition to symptoms of depression. The disorder develops in about 15 percent of people with major depression. Because of its symptoms, people with this disorder may not accurately judge the consequences of their actions and are therefore at risk for killing themselves. For these reasons, people with psychotic depression need immediate medical attention and probably require hospitalization.

Atypical Depression

People with atypical depression have a mix of symptoms, some typical of major depression and some atypical. For example, they may feel hopeless, discouraged, and self-critical like people with major depression. Yet they may eat and sleep more than usual, often gain weight, and usually feel worse in the evening than in the morning. By contrast, most depressed people lose their appetites, have trouble sleeping, and feel worse in the morning. Atypical depression also differs from major depression by usually being chronic (long-lasting) rather than being broken into episodes. Atypical depression usually begins in adolescence and may affect more women than men. People with atypical depression are generally treated with antidepressant medication, psychotherapy, or a combination of both treatments.

Postpartum Depression

Postpartum depression is marked by the same symptoms as major depression, and some researchers believe postpartum depression may be a form of major depression. This illness develops in approximately 10 percent of new mothers. Many different kinds of women get postpartum depression, but it is most likely to affect women who have already had major depression or a certain type of mild depression. Other factors also influence whether a woman will develop postpartum depression. According to some statistics, the woman who is most likely to get the disorder has had a difficult pregnancy or delivery, has an unhappy marriage, and gets little support from her friends, family, or neighbors.

Postpartum depression is more severe, prolonged, and disabling than the normal, temporary "blues" that affect most women the first few days after giving birth. If untreated, postpartum depression can last for months or even years, yet many women fail to seek help. Instead, they typically blame themselves for feeling sad at a time when they are expected to be happy. While it is normal to have fluctuations in mood after the delivery of a child, protracted depressed mood, lack of appetite, or sleep disturbances not related to the awakenings of the infant merit an evaluation by a physician. Postpartum depression may be treated with any one or a combination of the following: talk therapy, group therapy, and antidepressant medication.

Postpartum Psychosis

In rare cases, postpartum depression can develop into a more serious condition called postpartum psychosis. This illness occurs in 1 or 2 out of 1,000 new mothers. Its symptoms include hallucinations, delusions, and suicidal thoughts. Women who are experiencing postpartum psychosis need immediate medical treatment and probably require hospitalization.

Premenstrual Dysphoric Disorder

Premenstrual dysphoric disorder is a cyclic illness that affects some 3 percent to 5 percent of menstruating women. Women with this illness feel deeply depressed and/or irritable for a week or two before or during menstruation, and their symptoms are much more severe than those associated with premenstrual syndrome (PMS). Treatment for premenstrual dysphoric disorder may include exercise, various types of psychotherapy, and/or antidepressant medication (see Chapter 6).

DYSTHYMIA

Dysthymia, sometimes called minor depression, is a long-lasting form of depressive illness that is marked by a persistent lack of joy. If you have dysthymia, you are gloomy all or most of the time. You may be unable to remember ever feeling cheerful or excited. People with dysthymia often describe themselves as having been "depressed since birth." You probably lack a sense of humor and find it hard to have fun. Worry and guilt dominate your thoughts, and you tend to be withdrawn and lethargic. You may need 9 hours or more of sleep, or you may suffer periodic bouts of insomnia. No matter what the circumstances of your life, you feel like a failure. You tend to criticize yourself and others. Complaints come easily to your lips. You may even have thoughts of suicide (though not any active plans, which are signs of major depression). Yet, you may be devoted to your work and may be dependable and self-sacrificing at the office. You may feel this way all the time, without any break at all, or your symptoms may briefly lift from time to time.

Characteristics of Dysthymia

Doctors typically diagnose dysthymia in a person who has been feeling depressed nearly all day and every day for more than 2 years with no more than a 2-month period without symptoms and if the symptoms seriously bother the person or disrupt his or her life. In children and adolescents, an irritable mood on most days for at least 1 year may be a sign of dysthymia. Other defining symptoms include at least two of the following:

- Poor appetite or overeating
- Problems sleeping or oversleeping
- Low energy
- Low self-esteem
- Poor concentration or difficulty making decisions
- Feelings of hopelessness

These symptoms seriously disrupt the life of a person with dysthymia. Your doctor will rule out dysthymia if you have ever had mild or severe mania, if your symptoms arise only during another mental illness, or if you feel this way as the result of substance abuse, prescription medication, or physical illness.

Dysthymia tends to last for many years. Sometimes it continues through a person's lifetime. Because this illness is so persistent, it can cause great disruption. Young people with dysthymia may find it hard to concentrate, and their schoolwork may suffer. The gloom fostered by dysthymia also often leads to marital tension. Some people with dysthymia commit suicide.

Dysthymia can also deepen into a more severe form of depression. As many as 50 percent of people with dysthymia later develop major depression or bipolar depression. Children with dysthymia are particularly likely to do so. This change can happen so gradually that you do not notice the worsening of your mood. Some people with dysthymia experience episodes of major depression at the same time. This condition is sometimes called double depression.

Who Gets Dysthymia?

At some time, about 3 percent of the US population will have dysthymia. Some researchers think the disorder may be even more common because it can easily go unnoticed and untreated. Among adults, the disorder affects two to three women for every man. Dysthymia may begin in childhood and adolescence. If you have dysthymia, you probably have another disorder, psychiatric or physical. You may be likely to have phobias, anxiety, or a personality disorder. Physical illnesses that can accompany dysthymia include multiple sclerosis, acquired immunodeficiency syndrome (AIDS), and hypothyroidism. In addition, people with dysthymia may abuse alcohol or other substances in an attempt to relieve their sadness. Children and adolescents with anxiety disorders, mental retardation, or attention-deficit hyperactivity disorder (ADHD, a condition marked by lack of attention, impulsive behavior, and hyperactivity) may also have dysthymia that goes undetected.

Nobody knows what brings on dysthymia. At one time, doctors thought it was simply a personality type. Today, they suspect that some people may inherit a tendency to develop the illness because many people with dysthymia have relatives with other mood disorders. In addition, researchers have found that when one identical twin develops dysthymia, the other twin often does so also. In some cases, dysthymia may be the aftereffect of an episode of major depression. Another theory is that dysthymia may be linked to a malfunctioning biological clock. People with dysthymia often have unusual sleep cycles, indicating that abnormal circadian (day and night) rhythms may be at the root of their illness. (Possible causes of dysthymia are discussed in greater detail in Chapters 3 and 4.)

Treatment for Dysthymia

There is no guaranteed cure for dysthymia, but treatment may ease your symptoms and prevent them from getting worse. Dysthymia generally begins early in life, yet most people wait an average of 10 years before seeking help. You may delay seeking treatment because you see your constant bad mood as a part of life. But the earlier you talk to your doctor, the easier it will be to find relief. It is especially important that children with dysthymia see a doctor, because early treatment may prevent more severe mood disorders, school failure, and substance abuse later in life.

In the past, dysthymia was treated primarily with psychotherapy, most commonly psychoanalysis. Other talking therapies that treat the disorder are cognitive therapy, behavior therapy, and interpersonal therapy. Many doctors believe a combination of psychotherapy and antidepressant medication is probably the most helpful treatment for people with dysthymia.

Not everybody recovers from dysthymia. About 25 percent of people who seek treatment continue to struggle with some symptoms. But medication can improve your mood, even if it does not entirely remove your depression, and psychotherapy can give you the skills you need to cope with some of the effects of the illness.

See Chapters 5 and 6 for further information on treatments.

SEASONAL AFFECTIVE DISORDER

SAD is a type of depression that occurs only at certain times of the year. Most people with this illness typically feel lethargic and depressed during the winter but normal or unusually happy during the summer. Generally, the depression will set in during October and November and will lift during March or April. Some people experience SAD at other times of the year, especially if they work in a dark place, have vision problems, or live in a place that is frequently cloudy.

Characteristics of Seasonal Affective Disorder

If your energy plunges during the fall and winter, you may have SAD. During these months, you may feel exhausted and need more sleep than usual. Your appetite increases and you especially crave carbohydrates (starchy foods). Between 10 and 20 pounds may creep on. You may find it impossible to concentrate on your work or get anything done around the house. Sadness and anxiety will dominate your mood, and you may find yourself avoiding friends or family members. If you are a woman, you may find your mood worsening in the days immediately before your menstrual period begins. In children, irritability, school problems, and difficulty getting out of bed during the winter may be signs of SAD.

The depression of SAD typically lasts 5 months. Once spring returns, you feel as if you are coming back to life. Your energy rises, you drop the extra pounds you gained over the winter, and your mood returns to normal or you may feel slightly more exuberant than normal. Many artistic people with SAD find that spring is their most creative time of the year.

Who Gets Seasonal Affective Disorder?

An estimated 10 million Americans, or 6 percent of the population, have SAD. Another 25 million may have a milder version of SAD that is essentially a protracted dose of the winter blues known as subsyndromal SAD. The farther north you go in the US, the more common SAD becomes. For example, about 1.4 percent of people in Florida may have SAD at any given time, compared with 9.7 percent in New Hampshire. SAD affects about four times as many women as men and usually starts during a person's twenties.

SAD is not well understood. Some proposed explanations for the disorder include low levels of the hormone serotonin, fluctuating levels of the hormone melatonin, and abnormal circadian (day and night) rhythms. Some researchers believe that some people may inherit a vulnerability to the disorder. (Causes of SAD are discussed more fully in Chapter 3.)

Treatment for Seasonal Affective Disorder

Treatment for SAD typically begins with light therapy, in which you sit under bright lights for a period of time every day. In some cases, a doctor will suggest an antidepressant or a change in lifestyle during winter months. See Chapters 5 and 6 for further information on treatment.

Summer Blues

Some people experience a kind of backward SAD and feel depressed in the summer and normal or unusually cheerful in the winter. In the US, summer depression is only about one fifth to one quarter as common as SAD.

If you have summer depression, you probably lose your appetite and some weight, have trouble sleeping, and feel anxious and agitated during the summer. Once winter arrives, you feel normal or unusually cheerful.

Not much is known about summer depression. Some people feel better by traveling north to a cooler climate during the summer. This may mean that the depression is in some way affected by the brain's temperature. If you have summer depression, your doctor will probably suggest treating it with antidepressants or the mood stabilizer lithium (see Chapter 6).

BIPOLAR DEPRESSION

Bipolar depression—also known as bipolar disorder, manic depression, or manic-depressive illness—affects at least 2 million people in the US today. If you have bipolar depression, your mood swings between two emotional extremes, or poles—sadness (depression) and euphoria (mania). Between periods of these emotional extremes, your moods may be normal. But during the depressed phase of your illness, you will experience the same symptoms as people with major depression. You may experience periods of a milder and less debilitating form of mania known as hypomania, which are marked by heightened activity, sensuality, cheer, and self-confidence. During the manic phase, however, your mood will become abnormally elevated, expansive, or irritable. Energy, joy, and self-esteem may become dangerously unlimited and may give rise to delusions. These mood shifts may have little or no connection to day-to-day events, and the shifting symptoms you experience may prevent you from leading your normal life.

Doctors do not fully understand the cause of bipolar depression. But many believe that most people with this illness probably inherit a tendency to develop it, although their environment also plays a part in fostering the condition. (Causes of bipolar depression are discussed more fully in Chapters 3 and 4.) Bipolar depression has no cure but can be controlled with medication. Other types of therapy may also help you deal with the difficulties of this illness and help treat dangerous periods of mania.

Characteristics of Bipolar Depression

In Chapter 1 we saw how emotional moods can be seen as a rainbow, each distinct mood blending into the next. People with bipolar depression move across a wide portion of the spectrum of this rainbow during the course of their illness. How wide a portion depends on their form of the illness. Some swing between the extremes of severe depression and mania, an illness called bipolar I. Others bounce mostly between depression and hypomania, an illness called bipolar II. These swings across the spectrum of moods can cause real distress. They can significantly interfere with how well people function in their social or family lives, in their jobs, or in other important aspects of their lives.

The cycles of bipolar depression vary. In many cases, the illness starts with depression. Depression may alternate with mania over days, weeks, or months. Normal mood may return in some people between periods of mania or depression; others have several bouts of depression in a row, or several bouts of mania. Some people with bipolar depression have repeated periods of depression and only occasional episodes of milder hypomania. Others experience frequent mania but infrequent depression. About 10 percent to 20 percent of people with bipolar disorder experience only mania without depression. Still others experience depression and mania at the same time.

The feelings of bipolar depression vary enormously with each phase of the illness. During the depressed phase, you may experience many of the symptoms of depression described above. You may experience feelings of despondency and worthlessness or you may have difficulty in concentrating. By contrast, hypomania feels good. You feel lighthearted and your shyness disappears. Ideas shoot into your mind with great frequency. You feel infused with ease, power, well-being, and omnipotence. During mania, the most intense form of the illness, everything speeds up. Your ideas come fast, too fast, so you cannot concentrate. You cannot keep up with your thoughts, and your memory fails. You are irritable, angry, frightened, trapped, and out of control. All of these feelings, as different as they are, are part of bipolar depression.

Bipolar depression can be dangerous. Mania greatly impairs your judgment, making reckless behavior likely. If your illness is severe, you may completely lose touch with reality and experience a delusion. During the depressive phase, you are likely to feel suicidal. Of people with untreated bipolar depression, at least 15 percent kill themselves. For these reasons, you may be treated in the hospital during acute depression or mania.

Who Gets Bipolar Depression?

At least 1.2 percent of Americans have bipolar depression. Unlike other forms of depressive illness, bipolar depression is equally widespread among men and women. Although it can develop during childhood or old age, this illness usually begins during adolescence or young adulthood. Many people with bipolar disorder have other illnesses, and substance abuse is especially common. In some people, bipolar depression develops after several years of major depression.

If you have bipolar depression, you will probably have it for the rest of your life. Most people who experience one episode of the illness later suffer more episodes. About 80 percent of people with bipolar depression have four or more episodes over their lifetimes. Episodes may become more frequent and more difficult to treat over time.

Symptoms of Mania

At first glance, mania may seem like a positive state of mind. Its symptoms include an abnormally upbeat mood, a mind that teems with ideas, and a sense of being uniquely talented and attractive. But in mania, these positive feelings lead to inappropriate or harmful behaviors. You may ill-advisedly lecture your company's chief executive officer on how to increase profits. You may plunge into business deals you have no way of honoring. You may begin a sexual affair with a coworker, then suggest to your spouse or partner that the three of you set up a home together. In extreme mania, you may think the physical laws of the universe no longer apply to you—that if you need to get somewhere in a hurry, you can drive toward oncoming traffic without getting hurt.

Mania intensifies every aspect of your life. This fervor is more than a feeling. Chances are you will be more active than usual, working 16 hours a day, perhaps dancing in clubs every night and painting abstract art in your spare time. You probably find such intensity highly satisfying, but your mind cannot sustain it forever. As mania progresses, your mood becomes wilder and less predictable. Your extreme joy may collapse into irritability. Any form of frustration becomes unbearable. You may indulge in outbursts that frighten other people. Rage may overwhelm you, especially if others try to restrain your behavior or rebuff your excessive social demands.

Eventually, most episodes of mania subside into severe depression. Suddenly, the effects of your actions may become clear and chilling. Your spouse or partner may have left you because you were unfaithful while manic. You may be deeply in debt. Your employer may be waiting for results of an ambitious project that you cannot possibly complete. At this point in the free fall from mania into depression, many people become suicidal and must be hospitalized.

If you are manic, you may not recognize the symptoms of

mania in yourself. A lack of insight is the hallmark of mania. You may deny being ill and refuse medical treatment. At first, you may not appear ill, especially to people who do not know you well. They may find your boundless energy and optimism contagious. Even some doctors may be swayed and may fail to diagnose your mania. Somebody who knows you well, however, will probably see that your mood is abnormal. It may fall to that person to insist you receive appropriate treatment. You are likely to resent his or her intervention. If you become oblivious to reality and become dangerous to yourself or others, you may need to be hospitalized against your will.

As with depression, mania cannot be identified by a laboratory test. Instead, doctors look for a specific pattern of symptoms. Like depression, mania is a syndrome, meaning it is characterized by a collection of symptoms that occur together. Perhaps because the symptoms of mania are so flamboyant, mania appears to be diagnosed more readily than depression. Even so, researchers suspect that up to one third of people who experience mania may receive no treatment.

The main sign of mania is an abnormally elevated, expansive, or irritable mood. This buoyant feeling must persist for at least a week to qualify as mania. In some cases, however, it will be so extreme that the manic person will be hospitalized after a shorter period of time. An unusually happy mood may be a sign of mania if it is accompanied by at least three other symptoms, and an excessively irritable mood may be manic if it occurs with four or more other symptoms from the following list:

- Inflated self-esteem or grandiosity (overestimation of your importance)

- A sharp decrease in the need for sleep
- A compulsion to talk more than usual or never stop talking
- High-flown or racing thoughts
- A tendency to be easily distracted by something trivial or irrelevant
- Rapid physical movements and notably increased activity in any area of your life, including your social, work, school, or sexual life
- Excessive involvement in activities that are likely to have bad consequences, such as unlimited spending

Mania will be diagnosed only if these symptoms are so severe that they prevent you from functioning normally at work, in social situations, or in your relationships with other people. At times, mania appears shortly after certain treatments for depression, such as following antidepressant therapy. Mania is not diagnosed in such situations. Symptoms of mania often appear suddenly and rapidly intensify over a few days.

CHANGES IN MOOD
Most manic people feel on top of the world. If you are manic, you probably feel a profound sense of joy that has no connection with the events in your life. Nothing can dent your self-confidence. Energy surges through you. You can accomplish an astounding amount in a short time. The world appears rich and exciting. Many thoughts amuse you, and you may be full of jokes and wisecracks. No event, no matter how distressing, can make you unhappy. This extreme joy is called euphoria. It may be expansive, extending to all other people or the world itself. You may long to embrace strangers or feel mystically at one with the uni-

verse. Socially, you may become intrusive, wanting to spend all your time with other people or calling your friends in the middle of the night.

Euphoria is especially common early in a manic episode. Later, this heady feeling is likely to turn into irritability, especially if others try to intervene. If events fail to develop as you planned, you may quickly move from laughter to hostility. Any attempt to thwart your desires may provoke uncharacteristic rage.

People who are manic exude optimism. You may think you are finally fulfilling your potential, creatively, socially, economically, professionally, and sexually. Self-esteem is exaggerated and completely out of keeping with true ability. For example, you might compose church music and insist that the choir should perform it, even though you have no musical ability. If you are manic, you truly believe nothing can stop you.

DISTORTED THINKING

Such unwarranted self-confidence may develop into a grandiose delusion, in which you think you have a special rapport with supernatural beings, television celebrities, or world leaders. As many as 75 percent of people with mania develop delusions. In this delusional state, manic people may feel immune to any kind of restraint, social or legal. This makes harmful behavior extremely likely. In severe mania, people may hear voices that are not really there. The voices may be heard continuously or occasionally, and they may or may not address the ill person by name. In some cases, the voices will serve to bolster a grandiose delusion. For example, a manic person may hear instructions on how to save the world from nuclear war.

Mania may also heighten your senses, so that ordinary experiences are intensely pleasurable. Food may taste better than ever before, for example. You may perceive colors and light in a new and interesting way.

Your thoughts will speed up during mania. Your mind may race from one idea to another, but you will find it hard to focus on any one of them. This flow of ideas will be impossible to shut off. The content of your thoughts may also be altered by mania. For example, you may be much more likely than usual to focus on yourself, especially your perceived abilities.

The speech of people with mania is highly unusual. During mania, you may speak without pause, raising your voice if anybody tries to interrupt. You may force your way into other people's conversations, oblivious to their attempts to ignore you. As mania progresses, your speech will become louder, faster, and more difficult for others to understand. The medical term for this behavior is pressure of speech.

Your speech may be full of rhymes, puns, jokes, and unusual word associations. You may coin new words or give old words new meanings. You may select words for their sounds—for example, because they rhyme—rather than for their meanings. This kind of word choice is known as a clang association. In extreme mania, your speech may be completely incoherent.

CHANGES IN BEHAVIOR

Mania is a time of intense energy. If you have mania, you may feel rested after only 3 hours of sleep. You may be able to keep going at a hectic pace for several days without sleeping at all. Despite skipping sleep, you are likely to rarely feel tired.

Distractibility is often a sign of mania. You may find it impossible to concentrate on one line of thought or topic of conversation. Instead, you may begin to talk about one subject, switch abruptly to a connected topic, then switch again to something connected to the second topic, and end up totally lost. Trivia easily diverts your attention. In addition, you may forget small details of ordinary behavior during mania, such as hanging up after a telephone call.

People with mania are hyperactive. It may be impossible to sit still, be quiet, or stop thinking. You may stride up and down a room for hours. Your enthusiasm for work and other activities may be boundless and unrealistic. For example, you may agree to attend several meetings and social gatherings on the same day that you intend to finish a difficult project.

Reckless behavior is typical during mania. If you are manic, you probably indulge in activities that seem fun but can harm you. For example, you may drive dangerously, enjoying the thrill of high speed. Mania warps your ability to judge the effects of your actions. It is not unusual for manic people to break laws they see as irrelevant. In some cases, manic people may behave so irresponsibly that their families are financially ruined.

People with mania are often impulsive. Early in mania, your actions may seem only a little odd. For example, you may wear pieces of clothing that clash with each other. As your mania progresses, you may suddenly decide to paint the house pink and immediately get to work. In some cases, this impulsiveness is combined with a sense of purpose. For example, you may believe you have a particular religious mission to carry out in North Korea or Oman. Your restraint may lessen as time goes by, and you may become threatening or violent. Some people who have threatened important figures, such as the president of the US, have been found to be manic.

Increased sexuality is common during mania. This, combined with the characteristic recklessness of mania, may lead you to engage in sexually promiscuous or dangerous behavior. In some cases, mania may be diagnosed and treated only after your spouse or partner discovers that you have been unfaithful. The medical term for the heightened sexuality of mania is hypersexuality.

Unreliability may be a sign of mania. Mania makes it difficult for you to distinguish between fact and fantasy. As a result, you may frequently tell lies and deceive others. A doctor who treats your mania will probably try to confirm through a third person any information you provide.

Problems in Diagnosing Mania

The symptoms of mania may vary from person to person, so diagnosis of the illness is sometimes difficult. Detecting mania can be particularly tricky in adolescents, because their symptoms may differ from those of adults. Signs of mania in adolescents may include substance abuse, suicide attempts, academic problems, moodiness or irritability, and fighting and other antisocial behavior. One of the problems with diagnosing mania in teenagers is that some of these same symptoms are also seen in healthy adolescents. Mania in teenagers is sometimes misidentified as schizophrenia, a serious mental illness characterized by disturbed thought. Mania is even less likely to be noticed or treated in younger children. And though mania is not common among children, it does exist. Children with mania may be incorrectly identified as having attention-deficit hyperactivity disorder (ADHD) (see page 39).

Another difficulty with diagnosing mania is that symptoms of the disorder can result from other problems as well. For example, similar behavior may result from the use of such substances as amphetamines, cocaine, or steroids. Or manic symptoms may be signs of physical disorders such as thyroid, liver, or kidney problems.

Given the sometimes disturbing behavior caused by mania, it is not surprising that mania often alienates other people. Before the illness is diagnosed and treated, your behavior may cause many hurt feelings. A coworker may be crushed when your enthralling tales of adventure abruptly turn into an attack on her abilities. The heightened sexuality of mania also has the potential to strain relationships and may make other family members see you as immoral. But manic behavior is a symptom of your illness and not a matter of free choice, though it may have very real and lasting consequences for you and for those who care about you. The sooner your symptoms are recognized and treated, the less destructive your mania will be.

Treatment for Bipolar Depression

Most people with bipolar depression can be successfully treated with medication. You will probably need to take medication for the rest of your life, although the types of drugs may change as you move between depression, normal moods, and mania. Without treatment, the risk of accidental or suicidal death is significantly higher than that of healthy people.

Many doctors believe psychotherapy can also help you, especially in accepting the idea of taking medication for the rest of your life. Researchers have found that people who participate in psychotherapy—whether individual, group, couples, or family—

are less likely than others to have a relapse. Bipolar depression cannot be cured, but early treatment makes it easier to postpone future episodes and blunt their severity.

Treatments for bipolar depression are discussed more fully in Chapters 5 and 6.

VARIATIONS OF BIPOLAR DEPRESSION

Several less common forms of bipolar illness exist. They include rapid cycling, dysphoric mania, mixed state depression, and cyclothymia.

Rapid Cycling

Some people veer between frequent episodes of depression, mania, and hypomania. Those who experience four or more episodes in a year have a rare form of bipolar illness called rapid cycling. Although lithium is the drug most commonly prescribed for rapid cycling, lithium often does not help. In addition, it is risky to use antidepressants during episodes of depression, owing to the risk of bringing on hypomania. Anticonvulsant medication may be prescribed instead, alone or with lithium. Rapid cycling may be fostered by an underactive thyroid gland, so you should receive a thyroid test and thyroid hormone replacement therapy if necessary.

Dysphoric Mania

Some people have a kind of mania that is much more subdued than ordinary mania. This type of illness is called dysphoric (or unhappy) mania. People with dysphoric mania tend to be younger, more severely ill, and have a long history of bipolar depression. Treatment of dysphoric mania may also be difficult, because it may not respond to lithium. In general, an anticonvulsant medication alone or with lithium is used to treat dysphoric mania.

Mixed State Depression

People who are severely ill may experience depression and mania at the same time. These people are said to be in a mixed state. Much remains to be learned about mixed states. One theory holds that this is a transitional phase between depression and mania in which some people remain stuck. People with this form of bipolar depression may not respond well to lithium or antidepressants. Instead, some doctors recommend anticonvulsant medication.

Cyclothymia

Cyclothymia, also called cyclothymic disorder, is a milder but more lasting form of bipolar I disorder in which a person swings between hypomania and mild depression. People with cyclothymia have short, irregular bouts of depression and hypomania that last for days rather than weeks. These moods can switch rapidly, so that you may wake up in a different mood than you had the night before. These symptoms can be very distressing, impairing you or limiting how well you function in your job, in your social life, or in other areas.

To be diagnosed with cyclothymia, adults must have short, irregular episodes of depression and hypomania for at least 2 years with no more than a 2-month period without symptoms.

Children and adolescents must have these symptoms for 1 year with no more than a 2-month break. Also, you must not have experienced the severity of a manic episode during the first 2 years of your illness. Cyclothymia often develops in people between the ages of 15 and 25. It may be mistaken for hyperactivity or for a personality disorder. It is more common in women than men. Most people with cyclothymia find that lithium helps them. Much remains to be learned about cyclothymia and how to treat it effectively.

IS MY DEPRESSION LIKE YOUR DEPRESSION?

The many forms of depressive illness are all very different. Yet each brings feelings of sadness, either all or some of the time. Some researchers have wondered whether the experience of depression is always the same. For example, if I have major depression and you have bipolar depression, is the sadness we feel the same? Researchers have also wondered whether the depression different people feel results from the same processes in the brain.

Most people with depressive illness never feel manic—about two thirds of people diagnosed with clinical depression have periods of depression only. The other one third also experience mania. However, of the people who at first get only depression, between 10 percent and 15 percent will eventually develop hypomania or mania. Because depression sometimes develops into mania, some researchers think the same process brings on both major depression and bipolar depression. The bipolar illness, according to this theory, is simply a more extreme result of that process. Other experts think depression and mania are two extremes on a continuum of human emotions. Most experts believe, however, that major depression and bipolar depression are completely different illnesses, even if they both bring times of sadness.

3

Major Causes of
Depressive Illness

The causes of depressive illness are complex and only partially understood. At one time, doctors thought depression resulted primarily from troubled thoughts or emotions. Suppressed anger, for example, was seen as one of the possible causes. Today, however, most doctors and researchers believe that there are three primary causes of depression—biological, genetic (inherited), and emotional and/or environmental—and that a combination of factors contribute to the illness.

Biological causes include changes in the chemistry of the brain or fluctuations in the body's secretion of hormones. Genetic causes result in an inherited vulnerability to depression. Emotional and/or environmental causes include stressful emotional situations, such as the lack of loving parents or the death of a parent during childhood. Depression may develop from the inter-action of biological, genetic, and emotional and environmental factors. For example, if one of your parents has depression, you may have inherited a vulnerability to the illness (a genetic factor). This vulnerability may affect the way your brain responds (a bio-logical factor) to the stress of losing your job (an environmental factor).

Sometimes symptoms of depression result from a physical ill-ness, as a side effect of prescription drugs, or as an outcome of substance abuse. Depression from these causes generally lifts when the physical illness is treated and good health returns. These secondary causes are discussed in Chapter 4.

BIOLOGICAL CAUSES OF DEPRESSION

The Brain and Depression

In trying to find a biological cause for depressive illness, many researchers are looking at how the brain functions in depressed people. The brain is our body's command center. It controls our thinking, emotions, behavior, movements, and body functions. You may not be interested in all the details of how the brain works, but the real point of research in this area is to develop medications that treat areas of the brain affecting depression.

The brain carries out its commands through the work of chemicals called neurotransmitters. These chemicals help carry a command or message through the brain's network of special nerve cells, called neurons. Neurons are organized into areas of your brain that specialize in different kinds of activities. For example, one area controls your speech, while another region controls your posture. Researchers of depressive illness are especially interested in a part of the brain known as the limbic system. The limbic system regulates your emotions, such physical drives as sexual desire, and your response to stress.

The limbic system is made up of several different structures. One important structure is the hypothalamus, a small area at the base of the brain. The hypothalamus is a control center that affects many aspects of our lives: appetite, sleep, sexual desire, body temperature, reaction to stress, and the timing of many other functions. In addition, this region of your brain regulates the pituitary gland, which controls many important hormones. Other parts of your limbic system include the hippocampus and the amygdaloid complex, which help you to interpret and act on emotions. The activities of the limbic system are so far-reaching that a problem in any aspect of its communication network, including the work of the neurotransmitters, could affect you in any number of ways, including altering your mood, behavior, and sleep patterns.

HOW THE BRAIN WORKS

To understand how changes in the supply of neurotransmitters may lead to problems in the brain, we need to take a look at the brain's structure. Your brain contains between 10 billion and 100 billion neurons. As you think and feel and act, your neurons transmit messages throughout your brain. The messages travel in the form of electrical impulses at incredible speed—taking less than $1/5,000$ of a second to zip from one neuron to another. This speed allows the brain to react quickly, making you laugh at a joke or cry out in pain before you consciously think to do so.

Your brain's constant activity is possible only because your neurons are highly specialized to transmit and receive messages. Each neuron consists of a cell body; a long, thin fiber called an axon; and a set of shorter, branching fibers called dendrites. Whenever a message passes through your brain—whether to smack your lips over pizza or to fantasize about a trip to the Bahamas—many nerve impulses jump from one neuron to the next. First, a neuron picks up the nerve impulse with its dendrites. Then, the nerve impulse charges through the cell body and down to the axon. From there, it leaps to a neighboring neuron.

This constant communication in the brain relies on a complex, tangled network of neurons. Every neuron has numerous dendrites to pick up messages and each has as many as 1,000 branches at the end of its axon to forward messages. Because of this, there are more possible connections between neurons than there are atoms on the planet Earth.

Scientists once thought that the connections between neurons were fixed at birth and never affected by experience. Today, scientists have learned that events in our lives—the amount of nurturing we receive or do not receive as infants, for example—have a great impact on how many of these connections are created. As you master new skills and feel new emotions, your network of neurons constantly forms new connections. For that reason, the connections between the neurons in your brain are unique.

Although neurons are connected in the sense that they communicate, they do not actually touch each other. Instead, there is a tiny gap, called a synapse, between each neuron. It is the job of the chemical messenger to transmit or carry a message across the synapse, hence the name *neurotransmitter*. But before neurotransmitters can do their work, the message must change from an electrical impulse to a chemical one. This change occurs after the message travels through the neuron and reaches its axon. The axon releases neurotransmitters to carry the message across a synapse to another neuron. Once the nerve impulse reaches the next neuron, it changes back into an electrical signal. This same transformation, from electrical signal to chemical signal and back to electrical signal, occurs again and again with every thought and action.

When your neurotransmitters carry a nerve impulse from one neuron to another, they do so in an orderly way. Each neurotransmitter has a distinctive shape, which allows it to dock at a special site on a neighboring neuron, much as a lock fits a key. The docking site is called a receptor. These sites can accept only a certain kind of neurotransmitter, but neurotransmitters can fit into several types of receptors.

After the neurotransmitter crosses the synapse and docks at a receptor, it makes one of two things happen. Depending on the message from the neurotransmitter, the nerve impulse either continues on its way or stops right there. The neurotransmitter remains docked at the receptor while the second neuron reads its message and decides whether to continue the nerve impulse.

As soon as its job is done, the neurotransmitter pulls away from the receptor. When it floats back into the synapse, your brain removes it. It does so in one of two ways. First, it may break up the neurotransmitter with a substance called monoamine oxidase. Or the neuron that originally launched the neurotransmitter may pull the messenger back in. This process is known as reuptake.

CHEMICAL MESSENGERS AND DEPRESSION
Scientists estimate that people have hundreds of neurotransmitters, but only about 30 have been identified. Of those 30, scien-

tists have found links between depression and the activity of three main neurotransmitters: norepinephrine, serotonin, and dopamine. Scientists call these neurotransmitters the biogenic amines. Other neurotransmitters may also contribute to depression.

Norepinephrine, serotonin, and dopamine are active in the brain areas that control activities that go wrong during depression. Each neurotransmitter operates primarily in a specific brain area. Your brain has millions of connective circuits, or pathways, running between its neurons. Of these, only a few specific pathways contain norepinephrine, serotonin, or dopamine.

Norepinephrine, for example, operates in a pathway that winds through the brain's pleasure centers, the hypothalamus and the limbic system. Together, these regions control our emotions; our physical drives such as appetite, sleep, and sexuality; and our reaction to stress. Norepinephrine is also concentrated in parts of the brain linked with fear and memory. Serotonin follows a similar pathway but originates in certain cells that may play a part in agitation and sleep. Dopamine is active in an area of the brain associated with emotions. Between them, these three neurotransmitters travel on pathways reaching many parts of the brain that control activities disrupted by depression and mania.

Once scientists began to understand how neurotransmitters helped the brain communicate, they put forth several theories on how the supply of neurotransmitters could affect a person's mood. These theories were based on the fact that antidepressants can ease depression in some people, and they apparently work by adjusting the supply of certain neurotransmitters in the brain. Two types of antidepressants, for example, increase your brain's level of norepinephrine. One type, known as tricyclic antidepressants, prevents the reuptake of norepinephrine. Another type, called monoamine oxidase inhibitors (MAOIs), stops the breakdown of norepinephrine in the synapse. Because both types of antidepressants boost the brain's concentrations of norepinephrine, an early theory suggested that too little norepinephrine caused depression, while too much norepinephrine caused mania. (See Chapter 6 for more information on types of antidepressants.)

However, researchers have shown that the answer to depression is not simple. They have found that some depressed people have high levels of norepinephrine. Also, not all depressed people feel better after an antidepressant increases their levels of norepinephrine. When people did respond to antidepressant medication, they usually did so after several weeks, even though the medication boosted their norepinephrine immediately. Obviously, the role of norepinephrine in depression is more complex than originally thought.

The neurotransmitter serotonin is also involved in depression. Researchers have found low levels of serotonin in some severely depressed people, including some who were suicidal. Therefore, some antidepressants work by increasing serotonin rather than norepinephrine. Here again, however, the link between low levels of serotonin and depressive illness is unclear, as some depressed people have too much serotonin.

Dopamine levels also change during episodes of the illness, rising during mania and falling during depression. Medication that reduces dopamine, such as the blood pressure medication reserpine, sometimes causes depression. Depression also results when such physical illnesses as Parkinson's disease reduce the supply of dopamine. (See Chapter 4 for information on physical causes of depression.)

Neuropeptides have characteristics of both hormones and

neurotransmitters. They work with neurotransmitters to make neurons more or less receptive to the brain's message. One type of neuropeptide is the group of chemicals called endorphins, which can control the brain's perception of pain and response to pain. Some people with minor depression have low amounts of some endorphins. The amino acid called GABA (gamma-amino-butyric acid), another neurotransmitter, also has been linked to depression. GABA helps to control the flow of nerve impulses by blocking the release of other neurotransmitters, such as norepinephrine and dopamine. GABA reduces anxiety when released in the body, and low levels of GABA have been discovered in some depressed people.

Researchers are uncertain exactly why changing levels of neurotransmitters can lead to depression. Part of their uncertainty results from the difficulty they have in studying these substances. Each neurotransmitter occurs in minute quantities, is found only in specific parts of the brain, and is quickly removed once its job is done. Because the neurotransmitters disappear so quickly, there is no way to directly measure levels of them in the brain. Instead, scientists measure levels of substances that are left over after the brain uses a neurotransmitter. These substances, called metabolites, are found in such body fluids as urine, blood, and cerebrospinal fluid. By measuring the change in the levels of certain metabolites in the body, scientists gauge the change in the levels of neurotransmitters in the brain.

Researchers are also uncertain whether depressive illness results from or causes changes in the level of certain neurotransmitters. Some researchers think it works both ways. According to these researchers, the chemistry of your brain affects your behavior and your behavior affects your brain chemistry. For example, repeated hardships may alter your brain chemistry, making you act in a depressed way. But if you change that depressed behavior by learning how to cope with stress, your brain chemistry may change and may ease your depression.

OTHER LINKS TO DEPRESSION

Neurotransmitters are not the only suspects in depressive illness. Some researchers think that receptors, the neuron's landing docks, also play a role. One theory suggests that depressive illness develops when one type of receptor is broken, even though the others are working well.

When your brain chemistry changes, your receptors may be altered as well. Some researchers think this may explain how anti-depressants work. For example, if an antidepressant increases the amount of a particular neurotransmitter in your brain, your receptors may respond by becoming less sensitive to that neurotransmitter. Antidepressants alter two types of receptors for norepinephrine. They make these receptors less sensitive or less abundant. If antidepressants do work by changing your receptors, this adjustment would take time. This probably explains why most antidepressants take effect only after about 2 weeks.

Some researchers are attempting to explain depressive illness by examining what happens inside a neuron after it receives a chemical message. Once a neurotransmitter docks at a receptor, a series of complicated reactions takes place inside the neuron. Substances in the wall of the neuron split into smaller compounds, which in turn ignite activity inside the neuron. According to one theory, these compounds act as "second messengers," carrying messages from the neurotransmitters to the neuron's center, or nucleus. This second messenger system is slowed down by lithium, a medication that subdues mania; thus, some researchers think a breakdown in the second messenger system may cause mania.

Hormones and Depression

While some researchers seeking a cause of depressive illness have focused on brain chemistry, others have focused on the activities of the endocrine system. The endocrine system helps your brain regulate many of your body's activities. It consists of tiny organs called glands, which manufacture and release chemicals called hormones into your blood. Hormones control many of the body's physical processes, including sexual development and how you react to stress. Hormones travel through your blood to various parts of your body, where they cause changes to occur. A significant number of depressed people have abnormal amounts of certain hormones in their blood, even though their glands are healthy. Some researchers think these hormonal irregularities may explain some of the symptoms of depressive illness, such as disturbed sleep, appetite changes, and irregular menstrual periods in women, since hormones are involved in all of these functions. In addition, people suffering from certain endocrine disorders sometimes experience depression. And, in some people with depression, the endocrine system develops problems even though their glands are healthy.

Hormonal irregularities in depressed people are especially intriguing because they may be linked to the fluctuations in brain chemistry found in depressive illness. Your brain and your endocrine system are connected at the hypothalamus. The hypothalamus controls many of your body's activities, including appetite, sleep, and sexual desire. It also controls your master gland, the pituitary gland, which regulates the secretion of hormones from many other glands. In running your endocrine system, your hypothalamus uses some of the same neurotransmitters that have been linked to depression—norepinephrine, serotonin, and dopamine. These neurotransmitters all play a part in the timing and regulation of hormonal secretions.

THE EFFECT OF CORTISOL

About 50 percent of depressed people have too much of the hormone cortisol in their blood. Cortisol is released by your adrenal glands, which are located near your kidneys. Adrenal glands help you react to stress. The high amounts of cortisol in some depressed people are thought to be linked to their depression because their cortisol levels typically fall back to normal as the depression lifts.

Normally, your endocrine system avoids excessive levels of any hormone through a complex feedback mechanism similar to that employed by a thermostat. Your body monitors the level of hormones in your blood. When a particular hormone reaches a certain level, your glands shut off secretion of that hormone. This mechanism does not work properly in many depressed people. A significant number of people with depression continue to secrete cortisol after it has reached excessive levels in their blood.

The faulty part in this thermostat mechanism seems to be the hypothalamus. In a healthy person, cortisol is secreted as the result of a series of chemical instructions. The hypothalamus releases hormones that stimulate the pituitary gland, which in turn secrete hormones that tell the adrenal glands to produce cortisol. Each step in the process involves hormones. First, the hypothalamus produces corticotrophic-releasing hormone (CRH). This hormone makes the pituitary gland secrete adrenocorticotrophic hormone (ACTH), which in turn causes cortisol to be released by your adrenal gland into your blood.

In healthy individuals, the hypothalamus also keeps tabs on how much cortisol you have in your blood. As the cortisol increases, the hypothalamus reduces its signal to the pituitary. As the cortisol decreases, the hypothalamus increases its signal to the pituitary. However, in many severely depressed people, the hypothalamus sends a constant signal to the pituitary, no matter how much cortisol is in their blood.

Particularly interesting to researchers is the relationship between cortisol and the activities of the brain in a person with depression. They have found that the more cortisol you have, the less of certain mood-altering neurotransmitters you have. This suggests that something controlling your cortisol levels—whether the hypothalamus itself or some other part of the brain—may influence your depression.

The timing of cortisol secretions is also abnormal in some depressed people. Healthy people secrete cortisol at specific times. Their levels of the hormone are highest at about 8 A.M. and 4 P.M. and lowest in the middle of the night. Some depressed people do not show the normal rise and fall of cortisol. They may have higher amounts of cortisol during the night, for example, or have a steady amount of cortisol at all times.

Doctors test cortisol levels with what is known as a dexamethasone suppression test (DST). In this test, you receive a dose of synthetic cortisol, or dexamethasone, before you go to sleep at night. The next day, your blood is tested for cortisol at 8 A.M. and 4 P.M. If you are healthy, your cortisol levels will first drop and then gradually return to normal as your hypothalamus reacts to the synthetic cortisol in your blood. In severely depressed people, about half will show an abnormal response in which cortisol levels are not suppressed or do not change following a dose of dexamethasone.

Not all depressed people show abnormal results on a DST. However, people who do show an abnormal DST result when depressed will show a normal DST when their depression has ended. If their DST result was abnormal, their doctor can give them a repeat DST to confirm that they are over the depression.

OTHER HORMONAL DISORDERS

Though much remains to be learned about the relationship between hormones and moods, they are clearly connected. Do abnormal hormonal levels cause your depressed mood, or does your depressed mood cause your hormonal irregularities? No one is sure.

Depression is sometimes a symptom of disorders or diseases of the hormone-producing organs; these illnesses include thyroid disorders, Cushing's syndrome, and Addison's disease. These are secondary causes of depression and are discussed in Chapter 4. Many researchers, however, believe that the hormonal abnormalities seen in some depressed people are caused by an underlying brain disorder that is also responsible for the depression.

Some depressed people show abnormal secretions of growth hormone, which is released by the pituitary gland. This hormone is released during sleep, and some depressed people have too little of it. Researchers believe there may be a connection between levels of growth hormone and depression because sleep disturbances are common during depression. Another hormone, melatonin, appears to be linked to seasonal affective disorder (SAD), the form of depressive illness that occurs during the winter (see Chapter 2).

The Importance of Sleep and Other Rhythms

Problems with sleep—too much, too little, or a disrupted sleep schedule—are well-known symptoms of depressive illness. But researchers are now coming to believe that problems with the biological mechanisms that regulate sleep may actually be a cause of depression.

Many of your body's activities follow precise, biological rhythms. Sleep is an obvious rhythmic activity—you generally need to sleep for about 8 out of 24 hours to feel well. This schedule can be altered slightly. For example, you may go to bed at 11 P.M. instead of 10 P.M. one night and still feel fine the next day. But any great disruption in sleep may make you miserable. If you start working a night shift, for example, and try to sleep when your body knows it is day, you may not feel well until your system adjusts to the new schedule.

Although you are probably unaware of them, many other physical processes—including your body temperature, blood pressure, and hormonal secretions—are also rhythmic, rising at certain times during the day and falling at others. Your body temperature, for example, fluctuates by about 3 degrees over 24 hours, hitting its highest point during the afternoon and falling to its lowest point when you are deeply asleep. These natural biological cycles are called circadian rhythms, meaning that they occur about once every 24 hours. The word *circadian* comes from the Latin words meaning "about a day." In many depressed people, such circadian rhythms as the sleep cycle are seriously disturbed. Some researchers think that these disrupted cycles are more than a symptom of depressive illness and may actually aggravate or even cause the disorder. The idea that mistimed circadian rhythms may cause depressive illness remains unproven. If correct, however, this idea would explain some of the rhythmic patterns peculiar to depressive illness:

- Most depressed people feel worse first thing in the morning compared to later in the day.
- Symptoms come and go, sometimes recurring at the same time each year.
- Some people feel more depressed at certain times of the year.
- Depression may worsen every 28 days in menstruating women.

Biological Cues

The timing mechanism that controls our daily rhythms is often referred to as a biological clock. Scientists are still learning about how this mechanism works and which parts of the brain play a role. Scientists do know that the mechanism is sensitive to light and regulates your inner rhythms according to cues provided by the world outside your body. The most important cues are day and night, because all of your circadian rhythms are keyed to the day–night cycle. Social cues include daily schedules and regular eating times. Other cues include clocks, noises, and artificial lighting. In a person with depressive illness, the timing mechanism may be disrupted. As a result, this theory states, certain biological events, such as the secretion of hormones, are thrown off their regular schedule.

RAPID EYE MOVEMENT SLEEP AND DEPRESSION

Sleep patterns are significantly disturbed in people with depressive illness. Many depressed people cannot fall asleep. Some wake up several times during the night. Some wake early in the morning and cannot go back to sleep. Others sleep for many hours yet never feel rested. In mania, the need for sleep almost disappears. All of these disturbances are rhythmic and may be caused by mistimed circadian rhythms.

Scientists have found that when depressed people do manage to sleep, their sleep is abnormal. A test called an electroencephalograph (EEG) is used to study sleep. An EEG measures and records the electrical waves that your brain emits, whether you are awake or asleep. Using EEGs, researchers have found that the sleep cycles of depressed people seem to run backward.

There are actually two kinds of sleep: the kind with dreams, called rapid eye movement (REM) sleep, and the kind without dreams, called non-REM sleep. Most of the night, healthy people have non-REM sleep. During non-REM sleep, mental activity slows down but does not stop. Your brain sends out slower but larger and larger brain waves. During REM sleep, these brain waves become small and fast, similar to those of a conscious person. Your eyes move rapidly. Dreams play across your mind. Your heartbeat and breathing become irregular, indicating that your nervous system is aroused.

Non-REM sleep is divided into four stages. When you first fall asleep, you enter the first stage. This sleep is light. Your brain waves are small and fast, and you can easily be awakened. After about half an hour, your sleep becomes deeper. As you fall more and more soundly asleep, you go through stages 2, 3, and 4 of non-REM sleep. The deepest sleep occurs in stage 4, when your brain waves are large and slow. This is the time when growth hormone is released into your body.

After more than an hour, you enter REM sleep for a short time, then fall back into non-REM sleep. For the rest of the night, you continue to switch between the two kinds of sleep. Researchers think that REM sleep and the deepest form of non-REM sleep (stage 4) may be the types of sleep we need the most.

Your sleep is also divided into 90-minute cycles. During each 90-minute period, you have some non-REM sleep and some REM sleep. At the beginning of the night, during the first 90-minute cycle, most of your sleep will be non-REM. For example, it might consist of 80 minutes of non-REM sleep and 10 minutes of REM sleep. But as the night goes on, each cycle consists of more REM sleep. The fourth cycle, for example, might consist of 30 minutes of non-REM sleep and 60 minutes of REM sleep. This is why it is often easier to remember a dream that occurs close to morning. This regular, 90-minute cycle implies that our biological clock's pacemakers control sleep.

In depression, this regular pattern of sleep is disturbed. Depressed people experience REM sleep much earlier in the night than healthy people. Doctors call this unusual sleep pattern shortened REM latency. These irregular sleep patterns also occur to a lesser extent in people who have recovered from depression and in the relatives of depressed people. Some scientists think such sleep patterns may be a sign that a particular person is prone to depressive illness.

Depressed people also have more REM sleep in the first part

of the night and less REM sleep in the end of the night. This pattern is the opposite of that found in healthy sleep. In addition, depressed people get less deep sleep. They may skip stages 3 and 4 of non-REM sleep altogether. This may explain why some depressed people feel tired no matter how many hours they sleep. People with depressive illness also have more eye movements during REM sleep, more trouble falling asleep, and more trouble staying asleep. Their sleep toward morning becomes very light and may be marked by many brief awakenings.

Another link between depressive illness and the circadian rhythms is the effect of lithium on the body's rhythms. Besides being a medication for mania, lithium is one of the few substances known to alter circadian rhythms. When taken by healthy people, lithium lengthens the body-temperature cycle, so lithium may curb mania in part by resetting circadian rhythms.

Another treatment for depression—a change in sleeping patterns—also points to a connection between the illness and circadian rhythms. Many depressed people feel strikingly better if they stay awake for one complete night. Others show improvement if they wake up before 2 A.M. and thus miss the second half of sleep. This improvement is remarkable but unfortunately short-lived. Scientists speculate that the improvement may come from being awake when certain circadian rhythms change course. They point out that your blood pressure, pulse rate, and body temperature all reach their lowest point after 2 A.M. and then start to rise again. Sleeping at a different time has also temporarily helped some people with bipolar depression.

HORMONAL RHYTHMS

Sleep is not the only circadian rhythm disturbed during depressive illness. Hormonal secretions, which also follow circadian rhythms, can also be disrupted. For example, the rhythmic secretion of the hormone cortisol is often thrown off in depressed people. The cyclic production of the hormone melatonin may also be disrupted. Melatonin is secreted by the pineal gland, a tiny organ near the center of your brain. Melatonin is involved in regulating the rest–activity cycle. (It appears to have other effects on the body, too, but these are not well understood.) In healthy people, melatonin is secreted during darkness and shuts off during daylight. Thus, levels of melatonin in your body rise during the night and fall during the day. Some researchers have found that this rhythm is absent in about three fourths of depressed people.

The melatonin cycle is also out of sync—rising during the day and falling at night—in people with bipolar depression and may remain out of sync even after symptoms subside. Melatonin is also believed to play a role in SAD. People with SAD typically feel depressed during the dark winter months, when levels of melatonin rise.

The connection between circadian rhythms and depressive illness may lie in the functions of the depressed person's brain. The same neurotransmitters involved in depressive illness, such as serotonin and norepinephrine, are important for healthy sleep.

GENETIC CAUSES OF DEPRESSION

For many years, doctors have known that depressive illness runs in families. Many people with major depression or bipolar disorder can name family members who also struggle with the illness. However, for a long time, there was no way to know for sure if people inherited a susceptibility to depressive illness or if the illness was caused by something in the environment. Today, researchers understand that depressive illness is to some extent inheritable. You may have inherited a vulnerability to depressive illness, just as other people may have been born with a tendency toward rheumatoid arthritis. You have not inherited the illness itself, however—only a tendency to develop it. A unit of heredity called the gene carries this tendency.

The Gene and Inheritance

A gene determines which features you inherit from your parents. Many of your traits—whether your eyes are blue or brown, or whether you are male or female—are determined by the gene for that trait. Every one of your body cells has between 50,000 and 100,000 genes, all made of a substance called deoxyribonucleic acid (DNA). Genes are found in the nucleus of the cell (the control center) on threadlike structures called chromosomes. All of your cells, except sex cells, have 46 chromosomes, and most genes occupy a certain place on a certain chromosome. In most people, the genes are arranged in a completely individual way. Unless you are an identical twin, nobody in the world has your exact genetic makeup.

Sometimes, people inherit one or more abnormal genes from their parents. These abnormal genes may lead to health problems. For example, people with hemophilia are born with a defective gene. As a result, their bodies are unable to produce blood clots when they bleed.

Depression in Families

Depressive illness is believed to be partly hereditary because research on families shows that some are more prone to it than others. Brothers, sisters, and parents of people with major depression are two to three times more likely than other people to develop the illness themselves. Close relatives of people with major depression are also 1.5 to 2.5 times more likely to have bipolar disorder. The fact that such close relatives are all susceptible to depression implies that the disorder is passed down from one generation to the next.

Bipolar depression, in particular, runs in families. About 50 percent of all people with bipolar depression have at least one parent with a history of depressive illness. If a parent has bipolar depression, there is a 25 percent chance that his or her child will also have some form of depressive illness. This chance of an offspring having depression rises to between 50 percent and 75 percent if both parents have bipolar depression. Brothers and sisters of people with bipolar depression are also 8 to 18 times more likely than other people to develop bipolar illness. In addition, these relatives are 2 to 10 times more likely to have major depression.

Much of the evidence pointing to a genetic role in depressive illness comes from research done on twins. Twins are useful to genetic researchers because identical twins have the exact same genetic makeup, but fraternal twins do not. While identical twins have all their genes in common, fraternal twins have only 50 percent of their genes in common, just like ordinary brothers and sisters. Suppose one identical twin has blue eyes. Because that trait is entirely determined by genes, the second identical twin would also have blue eyes. In the matter of eye color or any other trait that is entirely controlled by genes, the traits of identical twins will always be the same.

In studying depressive illness, researchers have looked at

identical twins to see if it happens that when one identical twin is clinically depressed, the other is also depressed. Then, they have compared depression in identical twins with that in fraternal twins. Researchers in the US, England, Germany, Norway, and Denmark have found that identical twins are much more alike than fraternal twins when it comes to depressive illness. When one identical twin is depressed, the other twin is depressed 76 percent of the time. When a fraternal twin is depressed, the other twin is depressed only 19 percent of the time.

These findings point to a strong genetic influence on depressive illness, but they are not conclusive. The identical twins who were studied by researchers grew up in the same home and were therefore influenced by the same environment. It could be that something in that shared environment fostered depressive illness. Also, researchers know that twins are greatly influenced by each other. They speculated that one twin's depressive illness could in some way have affected the other twin.

Research on adopted identical twins bolstered the case for a genetic role in depressive illness. Identical twins who were reared apart were both depressed 67 percent of the time. Again, this implied that depressive illness is to some extent inherited.

All of these findings strongly suggest that genes play a part in depressive illness. At the same time, they show that genes by themselves do not decide whether a person becomes depressed. Researchers believe that a person's experience, such as the emotional losses suffered during childhood, may affect a person's genetic vulnerability.

More evidence pointing to depressive illness as a genetic condition came from researchers in Belgium. They focused on adults with bipolar depression who had been adopted as children. Researchers found that the adoptees' biological parents were more likely to have bipolar depression than were the adoptive parents. This suggested that the genes shared by the biological parents and their children were more important than environment in promoting bipolar depression.

The Search for the Depression Gene

As part of the search for a link between depression and genetic inheritance, scientists have tried to identify specific genes for depressive illness. Different researchers have pointed to different genes, but no single gene has been shown to consistently affect depressive illness in all families. Many experts believe that particular genes may cause depressive illness in some families but not in others. Also, several genes may work together to produce depressive illness in some families.

In trying to find a specific gene for depressive illness, scientists use a process called gene mapping. In gene mapping, each of the 46 chromosomes has been assigned a number. Scientists try to locate a particular gene for a trait on a particular chromosome to determine which genes are responsible for which genetic illnesses. For example, an abnormal gene on chromosome 4 causes Huntington's disease, a severe disorder of the nervous system.

In mapping genes, researchers look for genetic markers— particular variations that are inherited along with a specific gene. The location of many genes—that is, on which chromosome they lie and where on the chromosome—is unknown. But researchers do know how to find certain variations on specific chromosomes, including those that probably lie close to the gene that influences depression.

Scientists first identified a gene linked to depressive illness in 1987. This gene, found on chromosome 11, was reported to carry the susceptibility to bipolar depression. Researchers located this gene after probing the genetic material of Amish people in Pennsylvania. This community of Amish people, who are members of a conservative Protestant sect that stresses withdrawal from the modern world, is taking part in an ongoing research project on depressive illness. The Amish are no more prone to depressive illness than is any other group, but for genetic researchers, their community is a natural laboratory. For example, the Amish maintain extensive family records; encourage large families, which are helpful to genetic researchers; and forbid the use of alcohol and drugs, which means depressive illness among them is rarely masked.

Researchers analyzed the genetic material of 32 Amish families who were prone to bipolar illness. They became convinced that a single gene made these families vulnerable to bipolar depression. Later, they announced they had found a marker for this gene on a particular part of chromosome 11. Therefore, it seemed that a gene in this location made people susceptible to bipolar depression.

These findings were later undermined, however, after researchers enlarged the group of Amish whom they were studying. These newcomers seemed to have an inherited form of bipolar depression but apparently did not carry the gene marker on chromosome 11. In addition, one person who became mentally ill also lacked the marker on chromosome 11. As a result of these findings, scientists now suspect that at least two genes in the Amish community control a tendency to develop depressive illness.

At the same time, researchers in the US and Belgium announced that a gene on the X chromosome made some people vulnerable to bipolar depression. The X chromosome helps determine your sex; women have two X chromosomes and men have one. Other researchers who tried to duplicate these findings, however, had mixed results. Scientists now think that the gene on the X chromosome may make only some families prone to bipolar depression.

Additional research has pointed to a role for other genes in manic depression. Scottish researchers studied 120 members of a family, including 11 people with manic depression and 16 with major depression. They found a particular variation on chromosome 4 in all of the people with manic depression and in 14 of those with major depression. A later analysis of 11 families prone to manic depression also found a statistical link between the illness and the variation on chromosome 4.

In the US, scientists investigated all 46 chromosomes in members of five Amish families prone to bipolar depression. They reported that genes found on chromosomes 6, 13, and 15 may influence the illness.

Other researchers have pointed to a connection between a gene on chromosome 18 and a predisposition to manic depression. In the US, scientists studied 22 families that among them had 167 members with manic depression or major depression. In 8 of the families, variations were found at the same location on chromosome 18. Genes on that part of chromosome 18 influence functions that often go wrong in depressive illness. For example, a gene in that area affects a protein that allows neurons to receive messages from neurotransmitters. Proteins are substances that are important in the building, maintaining, and repairing of cells. A second gene on chromosome 18 controls some of the body's stress hormones, which are often disturbed in depressive illness.

Much remains to be learned about genetic influences on depressive illness. It seems likely that one of a number of genes may make you vulnerable to depressive illness. But no research so far has drawn a definite link between a specific gene and a predisposition to depressive illness in all people. Some genes, however, may carry a predisposition in certain families. Some scientists believe that several genes act together to make you susceptible.

Even if you inherit a gene that makes you vulnerable, that does not mean you will definitely develop a mood disorder. According to one estimate, if you inherit a genetic vulnerability, you have between a 50 percent and a 70 percent chance of developing the illness. One consistent finding from all these genetic studies is that depressive illness is not decided entirely by your genes. Some doctors believe that genes decide about two thirds of your chance of getting depressive illness. This means that one third of your chance is probably decided by your environment. However, the specific environmental events that may cause this illness in vulnerable people are not clearly understood.

EMOTIONAL AND ENVIRONMENTAL CAUSES OF DEPRESSION

Long before such biological aspects of depressive illness as neurotransmitters, hormonal secretions, or circadian rhythms were studied, doctors knew that many outside events could affect your mind and emotions. Your relationships with others, upbringing, losses, and crises can all influence your state of mind. In reacting to these influences, your mind may develop a depressive illness. Researchers exploring the connection between the mind, outside events, and illness have put forward several theories about the causes of depressive illness. Some of these theories are psychological, focusing primarily on the workings of the mind. Others are psychosocial, examining the workings of the mind within the wider context of society.

Of course, sifting between the biological, psychological, and environmental causes of depressive illness is not easy. Scientists are learning that these causes are not separate but interwoven in a complex relationship. Abnormal brain activity can color your mind's reactions to the events in your life, ensuring that you see only the bad in every situation. By the same token, a crisis may trigger a stress reaction within your body, affecting your brain and leading to depressive illness.

When Stress Causes Depression

STRESSFUL EVENTS

The relationships among stress, your body's response to life's hardships, and depressive illness are complex. Most researchers agree that some people become clinically depressed after a stressful event. Often, such events are negative and traumatic, such as a job loss, the end of a relationship, or the death of a close relative. But positive events, such as getting a new job or getting married, cause stress, too. Many people with depressive illness can point to an event or crisis that preceded their illness and perhaps fostered it. Yet it is far from clear whether painful events by themselves directly cause depression. All people struggle with hurtful changes at some time in their lives, and the majority never develop depressive illness. And some people develop depressive illness even when everything in their life is going well. In some cases, depression follows a change that seems good, such as a job promotion or retirement to a milder climate.

Some doctors think stressful experiences do cause depressive illness, but only indirectly. For example, if a woman with a genetic predisposition to depressive illness watches her husband die after a sudden illness, she may develop major depression. In this woman, a traumatic event caused depressive illness, but only by acting in combination with her genetic vulnerability. Some researchers think stress plays little or no role in bipolar depression, which has a strong genetic component. Others say that a first episode of bipolar depression may be set off by a painful event.

The relationship between stress and depression is especially murky in long-lasting depression. A loss or crisis is more likely to precede a first or second episode of depression. After those initial episodes, however, subsequent episodes often occur spontaneously. Researchers are uncertain why stressful life events are more likely to precede the first episodes of depressive illness than the later episodes. But according to one theory, the first episode may lead to long-lasting changes in the chemistry of the brain. This theory, called the kindling-sensitization hypothesis, suggests that the initial episode kindles, or sparks, long-lasting (or permanent) changes in the brain's limbic system, making it more sensitive to future episodes. Because the first episode increases a person's vulnerability to depression, minor stressful events can more easily set off later episodes.

Researchers based the kindling-sensitization hypothesis on the behavior of animals in laboratory experiments. They have found that if they stimulate an animal's limbic system with an electrical current, the animal eventually develops seizures. In addition, the animal's brain changes so that it becomes predisposed to future seizures. Even after an animal has been left alone for many months, it will have a seizure if the current is applied again. Some of the animals have spontaneous seizures, especially if they are in the place where the current was originally applied. This shows that the seizures can be triggered by the animal's environment. Stress has also been shown to make the animals more sensitive to the current.

The kindling process would explain why anticonvulsant medication, normally given to treat recurring seizure disorders, is useful in treating depressive illness, particularly bipolar depression. If such kindling has a residual effect, it would also explain why stressful events make you vulnerable to depression, why episodes of depression tend to get worse over time, why later episodes start to come faster together, and why people with depressive illness gradually become prone to spontaneous relapses.

For some people, life's difficulties and depression are intertwined, with each constantly feeding the other. It may be hard to pinpoint which came first, a painful event or your anguished feelings. If you are depressed, you may be able to trace your illness to a particular hardship. At the same time, your depression is warping your view of everything in your life, including that hardship, so that you can see only the down side.

CHRONIC STRESS AND LEARNED HELPLESSNESS

Chronic stress—that is, difficulties that are present, day in and day out, over a long time—may also spark depression in some people. Depression may be set off by a constant struggle to fill multiple roles or by a change in the roles you are expected to fill. People with major depression or dysthymia often talk about ongoing problems in juggling numerous roles, such as having to act as a loving mother at home and an assertive corporate executive at work. Major life transitions, when your roles change dramatically, are particularly likely to foster depression. The times of such transitions include (1) late adolescence, when you may be pulling away from your family and trying to establish yourself as an independent adult; (2) middle age, when you may be adjusting to changes in fertility or virility as well as wondering whether you can still advance in your career; and (3) the years after retirement, when you may be struggling with a reduction in prestige or income after the end of your career.

A single painful event is also more likely to trigger depression if you are under chronic stress. This is especially true if the chronic hardships and the hurtful incident touch on the same part of your life. For example, if you are unhappily married, you may become clinically depressed after your daughter leaves home and moves far away. Chronic stress and difficult events are often interrelated. Together, they may trigger depression that the event by itself would not. For example, if paying bills is a constant stress factor, losing your job, which will only increase that type of stress, may be more likely to trigger depression.

Researchers are investigating exactly how stressful events cause depression. One theory is that people who experience repeated stress learn to feel helpless, especially when they have no control over the stressful situation; this learned helplessness is thought to lead to depression.

The learned helplessness theory is based on laboratory experiments in which animals were subjected to two kinds of electrical shocks. At first, the animals were exposed to shocks they could not escape. Then, they were exposed to shocks they could escape.

Animals who had received the inescapable shocks had trouble avoiding the escapable shocks. They had apparently learned that their efforts to escape were futile and they were helpless. These animals showed some behavior usually seen in depression. For example, they had trouble eating and sleeping. By contrast, animals that had not received inescapable shocks easily avoided the escapable shocks and did not have trouble eating or sleeping.

While studying the animals that had learned helplessness, researchers found that their brain chemistry had changed. Their receptors for the neurotransmitter norepinephrine had changed. Some receptors had become more sensitive to the neurotransmitter, and others had become less sensitive. Researchers then treated some of the animals that had learned helplessness with antidepressants. These animals quickly learned to avoid the escapable shock. Finally, some animals that had learned helplessness were taught how to stop the shocks by pushing a lever. Once the animals no longer felt helpless, their symptoms of depression lifted. After the depression eased, the animals' brain chemistry returned to normal. Researchers concluded from these experiments that experience does indeed affect brain chemistry and behavior. At the same time, behavior affects chemistry of the brain.

In humans, learned helplessness takes the form of negative and pessimistic beliefs about the ability to cope with life, based upon stressful experiences and failures in the past. When people attribute their failures to factors that are beyond their control, their risk for developing depression goes up.

Say you are an adolescent girl about 13 years old. You are at a point in your life when you may be particularly vulnerable emotionally. If you have a verbally abusive parent who continually tells you that you are stupid, you may come to believe it and doubt your ability to handle your own problems. This sense of helplessness may predispose you to develop depression. Some researchers believe that if you experience major stress, such as the death of a parent or the verbal abuse described above, early enough and strongly enough, your brain chemistry may be permanently changed, leaving you less able to handle stressful experiences.

When a Traumatic Event Leads to Depression

Researchers have found that single, painful events, such as divorce, illness, or a death in the family, are in some way linked to major depression. Most people with major depression report that something painful happened to them shortly before the onset of their depression. The loss of a spouse or partner due to death or divorce is the traumatic event most likely to trigger depression.

Depression is likely to result from random incidents that deprive you of any sense of control. Such crises include losing a job due to technological change, being caught up in a natural disaster, or being involved in a serious car accident caused by another driver.

In general, the more painful the event, the greater its potential to cause depression. Witnessing the death of a family member is therefore far more likely to trigger depression than is an argument with a neighbor.

Sometimes, the same sort of crisis can cause more emotional havoc for one person than for another. For example, men are more likely than women to become depressed after the death of a spouse. Some researchers think this is because the death of a wife leads to other losses for her husband. For example, a man may lose touch with his adult children after his wife dies, causing further emotional suffering and isolation. Such isolation may be less likely to happen to women, who tend to be more emotionally involved with their families and more likely to reach out to others.

Traumatic events can also affect your recovery from depressive illness. The more difficult your life, the longer your recovery is likely to take. If a particular event, such as the breakup of your marriage, triggered your depression, subsequent events that make the breakup even more painful will probably slow your recovery. For example, losing the custody of your children would probably set you back. On the other hand, events that make the breakup less painful, such as a positive and promising new relationship, are likely to speed your recovery.

In some cases, a normally painful event can help you feel better. For example, though the breakup of your marriage is painful, it might speed your recovery from depression if it resolves a different problem, such as your spouse's abusive behavior toward you. Sometimes, a harmful incident can help you recover in a roundabout way, by putting the event that triggered your depression into perspective. After surviving an automobile crash, for example, you may see the job loss that set off your depression as having little importance.

Some researchers think the link between depression and traumatic events is not clear-cut. They point out that a person's depression may cause a painful event, rather than the other way around. For example, if you are experiencing the poor concentration and confused thinking typical of depression, you may perform poorly in your job and risk being fired.

The Effects of Childhood Unhappiness

An unhappy childhood can lead to depression in adults. Severe difficulties during childhood—separation from a parent, family turmoil, mental illness in a parent, and sexual or physical abuse—occur more frequently in people with depression than healthy people. Some researchers think a difficult childhood is most likely to spark early-onset depression, in which a first episode occurs before the age of 20. Of all the single, painful events that are connected to depressive illness, the death of or separation from a parent before the age of 11 is the most significant.

Exactly how childhood suffering leads to adult depression is unclear. One theory is that unhappy children find it harder to cope with times of change, such as adolescence. Moving forward into adulthood, adolescents may find new roles particularly difficult. A different theory is that unhappy children are emotionally damaged in ways that make them prone to depression as adults. For example, unhappy children are more likely to feel powerless, have low self-esteem, and depend on other people to make them feel good. In turn, these personality traits may make adult depression more likely.

Other researchers point to the fact that a baby's brain continues to develop after birth and so is affected by the child's early experiences. The limbic system, the area of the brain that controls emotions, has a built-in flexibility at birth. This allows a baby to adapt to his or her environment. At the same time, that environment may be molding the child's brain, particularly its regulation of emotion.

Depression has been seen in infants separated from their mothers. During World War II, researchers noticed that children admitted to orphanages after their mothers died went through several stages of grief before succumbing to depression. At first, the babies protested and cried vigorously for their mothers. Then, they became extremely restless, presumably trying to attract the absent mother's attention. This protest was followed by despair, when the babies wept and were still. Finally, the babies became extremely withdrawn. This severe grief reaction was called anaclitic depression. *Anaclitic* comes from the Greek words meaning "leaning on."

Infant monkeys who are separated from their mothers go through the same stages of protest, despair, and withdrawal. Experiments have shown that these monkeys secrete greater amounts of the stress hormone cortisol into their blood during the protest stage. The greater the levels of cortisol during protest, the more profound their depression later. Remember that high levels of cortisol are found in the blood of about half of depressed people. Researchers do not know if this increase in cortisol is a sign that something is wrong or is the body's attempt to put things right.

The Depressed Personality

People of all personality types—outgoing, shy, deep-thinking, superficial, placid, and nervous—can develop depressive illness under the right circumstances. Your personality is the sum of your habits, traits, and experiences, influenced by your heredity and your environment. No particular trait or habit in your personality can cause depression. However, certain aspects of your personality may make you more prone to the illness. People who get depressive illness often set high standards for themselves, find it hard to relax, and may be reluctant to ask for help. If you are given to excessive worry, pessimism, or self-criticism, you may be more likely to become depressed. The same holds true for people who think they have little control over their lives. Depression is less common in people who are flexible, feel secure in their social setting, and find it easy to talk about their problems.

The Mind's Role in Depression

Physicians and psychologists, who study the mind and human behavior, have proposed various theories about the causes of depressive illness. The oldest theory was formulated by the Austrian physician Sigmund Freud during the late 19th century. Freud suggested that depression was caused by anger at others turned inward toward oneself. He drew a distinction between depression and normal grief, saying that depressed people are filled with guilt, self-reproach, and self-criticism, unlike healthy people in mourning.

Another theory is that depressed people have failed to absorb the loving attitudes of their parents into their own unconscious. Your unconscious, also known as the subconscious, is the part of your mind with thoughts, feelings, and ideas about which you are unaware. If people believe that their parents did not love them, they are filled with inner feelings of persecution and worthlessness. According to this theory, mania is used to protect the self by idealizing other people and denying any feelings of aggression toward them.

Some experts on depressive illness think depression comes from realizing the difference between your aspirations and what you have actually achieved in your life. When you see that you have not lived up to your ideals, you feel helpless and powerless. Others say depression results when you receive insufficient support from people you care about.

Still other experts think that depression develops when people routinely think negatively, criticize themselves, characterize themselves poorly, and otherwise undermine their self-esteem. A different theory is that people get depression when they do not receive the rewards they feel they deserve. Another idea is that depression stems from your perceived failure to live up to the expectations of other people. According to this theory, depressed people do not look inside for direction and strength but instead look to other people. Some psychologists think depression results when people cannot find meaning in life or lose the meaning they used to find.

When Other Psychological or Mental Disorders Occur With Depression

If you have another psychological disorder or mental illness, you may experience depression in addition to your other symptoms. Depression that occurs in the presence of another illness is called co-morbid, coexisting, or co-occurring depression. If depression develops after another psychiatric illness has already been diagnosed, your doctor may refer to it as secondary depression.

ANXIETY DISORDERS

General anxiety disorder is marked by feelings of dread, fear, or apprehension that are not appropriate reactions to events. If you have anxiety disorder, you may feel apprehensive and tense and may be unable to concentrate, or sleep well. In addition, you may have frightening dreams and occasional signs of fear, such as a pounding heart, sweating palms, trembling, or diarrhea. Depressive illness and anxiety disorder are closely related. About 30 percent of people with depressive illness also have symptoms of anxiety disorder.

In cases in which clear symptoms of both anxiety disorder and major depression exist, depression is often the underlying condition. However, people with anxiety disorders may develop depression as their illness progresses, especially if their symptoms are untreated. Your doctor can determine which illness is fundamental and thus should be treated first. There are several types of anxiety disorders, among them panic disorder and phobia.

Panic disorder is a kind of anxiety in which your body and mind experience sudden, intense fear. During this reaction, also known as a panic attack or anxiety attack, you may also experience physical symptoms, such as shortness of breath, sweating, trembling, dizziness, pallor, and stomach cramps. Panic disorder is linked with depressive illness. A large percentage of people with panic disorder go on to develop major depression within a few years. At the same time, between 10 percent and 20 percent of people with major depression may also have panic disorder.

Your treatment will depend on the nature of your panic disorder. If the panic occurs only during episodes of major depression, your doctor will probably treat the depression first. If you have suffered panic disorder in the past without major depression, you and your doctor will try to judge which is the most serious disorder. In making this decision, you will have to consider your family's history of each illness, how the illnesses have progressed, and how disabling each is.

A phobia is an anxiety disorder in which you experience an irrational fear of a specific object or situation. For example, you may fear spiders, heights, or other people. If you have a phobia, the need to face the situation you fear may bring on the symptoms of anxiety, such as a racing heart, sweating hands, rapid breathing, and a feeling of nausea. Phobias and depressive illness often occur together. Researchers say, for example, that more than 90 percent of people with an irrational fear of open spaces, called agoraphobia, develop depressive illness. If you have major depression and phobia, you and your doctor will decide which condition to treat first. This decision will be based on various considerations—in particular, which illness is the most disabling.

OBSESSIVE-COMPULSIVE DISORDER

Obsessive-compulsive disorder is characterized by intrusive and uncontrollable thoughts or impulses. Obsessions are persistent, unpleasant thoughts that you cannot ignore. Such thoughts may lead to compulsions, which are irresistible impulses to perform the same action again and again. A particular obsession may foster a certain compulsion. For example, you may become obsessed with a fear of germs and compulsively wash your hands again and again.

There are several links between obsessive-compulsive disorder and depressive illness. The illnesses share certain symptoms—such as excessive guilt, indecisiveness, low self-esteem, fatigue, and sleep problems—and often occur together. In general, if you have obsessive-compulsive disorder and depression, treatment will aim at easing the symptoms of both disorders.

PERSONALITY DISORDER

Personality disorder is an illness in which a person's emotional problems have affected and distorted the shape of his or her entire personality. Examples include paranoid personality disorder, in which the person is very suspicious in all personal relationships;

schizoid personality disorder, in which the person leads a very isolated and emotionally narrow life; and obsessive-compulsive personality disorder, in which a person obsesses over some idea and is very meticulous, rigid, and controlling. When depression occurs with personality disorder, the depression is generally treated first.

SCHIZOPHRENIA

The term schizophrenia is used for a group of severe emotional disorders that affect thinking, emotion, perception, and behavior. Schizophrenia alters a person's thought patterns, reactions to others, and behavior to such an extent that he or she undergoes a change in personality. People with schizophrenia show signs of fragmentation (disorganization) of the personality, experience delusions or hallucinations, and suffer significant thought disorders.

Manic depression is commonly misdiagnosed as schizophrenia, although this may be less likely to happen today than in the past. Some people suffering from mania experience symptoms similar to those of schizophrenia, such as delusions and hallucinations. People with mania who belong to ethnic minorities are particularly likely to be misdiagnosed with schizophrenia, especially African Americans and Hispanic Americans.

Bipolar depression and schizophrenia are so alike that some doctors think schizophrenia should be diagnosed only after bipolar depression has been ruled out. In trying to decide which illness you have, your doctor may prescribe lithium to see how you respond. Most people with mania find their condition improves with lithium, but fewer people with schizophrenia do. Also, your family history might help with your diagnosis. Both schizophrenia and bipolar depression tend to run in families but rarely occur in the same family. If you have relatives who suffer from bipolar depression, therefore, it is more likely that you have mania and unlikely that you will have schizophrenia.

Some people experience a confusing mix of symptoms, some typical of the bipolar depression and some typical of schizophrenia. For example, you may have the decreased need for sleep, increased energy, and racing speech typical of bipolar depression, yet you may experience a delusion that is not manic in its tone or content but seems characteristic of schizophrenia. Some doctors think that people with mixed symptoms have a type of manic depression rather than schizophrenia, but no one really knows for sure. For this reason, doctors often treat their patients with mixed symptoms for mania rather than schizophrenia.

EATING DISORDERS

Eating disorders, such as anorexia nervosa and bulimia nervosa, can also be connected to depressive illness. In anorexia nervosa, a person has a distorted body image and refuses to eat, possibly leading to extreme weight loss, hormonal disturbances, and in some cases, death. Bulimia nervosa is binge eating followed by attempts to purge the food, either through self-induced vomiting or laxative abuse. Both illnesses occur mostly in adolescent girls or young women.

The poor nutrition that is part of these disorders can itself cause depression. As many as one third to one half of people with eating disorders also suffer from depression. Some researchers have found that between 35 percent and 75 percent of people with bulimia also have mood disorders in the acute stage of their illness. In addition, between 50 percent and 75 percent of people who have eating disorders will go on to suffer from major depression later during their lifetime. Some researchers believe that eating disorders may be a kind of depressive illness because they cause similar changes to the chemistry of the brain. Also, similar hormonal abnormalities are found in people with depression and people with eating disorders. Other researchers think the depression is a direct result of the eating disorder.

If you have an eating disorder and depression, you and your doctor will have to decide which condition should be treated first. Typically, when the eating disorder is treated first, the depression lifts in most people as they return to a well-nourished state.

4

Other Causes of
Depressive Illness

The last chapter discussed the biological, genetic, and environmental or emotional causes of depression. These are the primary causes of depressive illness. But sometimes depression is a symptom of other disorders, not of emotional illness. In fact, major depression has an underlying medical cause in about 10 percent to 15 percent of cases. Depression that accompanies a physical illness or condition may be called co-occurring, coexisting, or secondary depression.

If you have depressive illness and a physical ailment, your treatment will depend on the precise relationship between the two conditions. If your depression is the biological result of a physical problem, your depression is likely to subside once the physical problem has been treated. If you have depressive illness and do not know its cause, chances are you do not have a serious medical condition, since most depressive illness does not stem from physical illness.

If your depression is a psychological reaction to such a serious physical illness as lung cancer, you and your doctor will probably decide to treat the depression in addition to the cancer. This treatment of secondary depression is a departure from the past, when many doctors saw depression as a reasonable reaction to a serious illness. Today, doctors realize that if your depression goes untreated, you may be less able to fight your physical illness and less likely to comply with its treatment. If you are physically ill and also have symptoms of depressive illness, in most circumstances your depression will be treated, too.

Symptoms of depression can result from a physical illness or disorder, from drug or alcohol abuse, or as a side effect of prescription drugs.

PHYSICAL CAUSES OF DEPRESSION

Hormonal Disorders

Disorders of the organs that produce hormones are the physical illnesses that most often cause depression. Thyroid disease, in particular, is often accompanied by depression. Thyroid disease is extremely common, especially among women. In some cases, depression and fatigue may be the first signs you notice of thyroid disease. There are two kinds of thyroid disease: hypothyroidism and hyperthyroidism. In hypothyroidism, the thyroid gland slows down and secretes too little hormone. In hyperthyroidism, the gland secretes too much hormone. Depression can be caused by either form of thyroid disease but is more likely to accompany hypothyroidism.

To rule out a sluggish thyroid as a cause of your depression, your doctor will measure your level of thyroid hormone with a blood test. Your doctor may also administer a thyroid-releasing hormone (TRH) stimulation test. First, a blood sample will be drawn to measure your baseline (normal for you) level of thyroid-stimulating hormone (TSH), the hormone that sends the thyroid into action. Then, you will receive a dose of TRH, the hormone that controls TSH production. Your blood TSH level will be drawn again 15, 30, and 90 minutes later. If your thyroid is healthy, blood samples will show your level of TSH has risen. If your depression is caused by a thyroid condition, your symptoms will lift once the condition is treated.

Diseases of the adrenal glands can also cause depression. Your two adrenal glands, which are found near your kidneys, are made up of two parts. The central part of the gland is called the medulla, which produces the stress hormones epinephrine and norepinephrine, which also act as neurotransmitters in the brain. The other part of the adrenal gland, called the cortex, produces hormones called corticosteroids. These hormones regulate your use of digested foods and your reaction to stress. Adrenal hormones also control the excretion of sodium and potassium by your kidneys and direct the development of your sexual characteristics early in puberty.

Depression is a common symptom of Addison's disease, in which the adrenal cortex gradually stops functioning. In fact, the depression may exist for some time before Addison's disease is diagnosed. In Cushing's syndrome, the level of corticosteroid hormones in your blood is too high. This usually happens as a result of corticosteroid medication taken for another illness. Sometimes it is the result of overactive adrenal glands, which are usually reacting to a tumor somewhere in the body. (If the tumor is in your pituitary gland, the condition is sometimes called Cushing's disease.) Severe depression is a common symptom of Cushing's syndrome. (Other symptoms of Cushing's syndrome include certain physical changes, including a round, red face, an obese upper body, and thin skin; weakened bones; hypertension; and edema.)

Hyperparathyroidism, a condition in which your parathyroid glands produce too much parathyroid hormone, may give rise to depression. The four parathyroid glands lie near the thyroid in the throat and secrete parathyroid hormone. This hormone increases the amount of calcium in the blood, a change to which your body is extremely sensitive. (Too much calcium, a condition called hypercalcemia, can cause excessive urination, tiredness, nausea, and vomiting. Severe cases can result in coma and even death if not treated.) Hyperparathyroidism is usually caused by a benign tumor in one of the four glands. About half of people with hyperparathyroidism also have depressive illness.

Depression may be a reaction to the physical complications of diabetes mellitus. In this disease, your pancreas, a gland that lies behind your stomach, produces little or no insulin, the hormone that regulates the use of a sugar in your body called glucose. This can cause eye, nerve, and kidney damage and other complications, which in turn can make a person depressed. There are two main types of diabetes mellitus. In type I, which occurs mainly in young people, the pancreas produces little or no insulin. In type II, which occurs mainly in people over 40, the pancreas secretes an inadequate supply of insulin. As many as one fourth of all people with diabetes mellitus also develop depressive illness.

Infectious Diseases

Infectious disease sometimes gives rise to depression, as a symptom of the disease or as a psychological response to illness. You may develop depression while still fighting one of these diseases or immediately afterward. Depression is often an early sign of mononucleosis, which results when the Epstein-Barr virus attacks your white blood cells. Symptoms of mononucleosis vary widely. You may feel as if you have a mild cold, or you may have a persistent sore throat, fever, swollen glands, headache, and weakness. If you do not develop depression early in mononucleosis, you may do so near the end of the illness. Depression may be the last symptom of mononucleosis to clear up.

Depression is also common with viral hepatitis, a liver infection caused by one of several viruses. Scientists have identified three main types of viral hepatitis, called A, B, and C. Viral hepatitis may be short-lived or chronic and recurring. Depression is more likely to be a symptom of hepatitis B or C than of hepatitis A, a very common and mild form of the disease. Your symptoms may be mild or severe but will generally include loss of appetite, nausea, vomiting, fever, joint pains, and yellowing of the skin. Depression may arise at any stage of viral hepatitis.

Viral pneumonia is an inflammation of the lungs caused by a virus. Depression or mental confusion often accompanies this illness, whose symptoms include a worsening cough, headache, muscle aches, and blue-tinged lips. Depression is likely to lift as the pneumonia clears up.

Cancer

Many people with cancer go on to develop major depression, though only a small percentage of people with depressive illness have cancer. Depression may be a symptom of the disease. Rarely, cancerous tumors can secrete the mood-regulating chemical serotonin, causing an imbalance that produces symptoms of depression. But depression can also develop as a psychological reaction to the pain, fear, and worry associated with cancer.

Depressive illness often accompanies cancer of the pancreas, an organ that lies behind the stomach and secretes juices that are essential to digestion. Cancer of the pancreas develops rapidly and is usually fatal within 3 to 6 months. Brain tumors are also among the cancers most likely to give rise to depression. In some cases, depression is the earliest or only symptom of a brain tumor.

Autoimmune Disorders

Some disorders of the immune system have been linked to depression. In autoimmune disorders, our immune system, which protects the body from disease, attacks the body's cells. One such disorder is systemic lupus erythematosus (SLE), in which the body's connective tissue becomes inflamed, damaging the skin, joints, and internal organs. Lupus can bring about mental changes, including depression. Some researchers have found that one quarter of people with lupus have mental changes, such as a decrease in short-term memory, shortly before or after their illness is diagnosed. In about 3 percent of these people, the mental changes are the only symptom.

Depression occurs in about 10 percent of people who learn that they have been infected by the human immunodeficiency virus (HIV), the virus that causes acquired immunodeficiency syndrome (AIDS). When HIV infection develops into AIDS, depression also develops in at least 30 percent of cases. Depression can result from the HIV infection itself, from other opportunistic infections that take advantage of the weakened immune system, from difficult treatments, or from the stress of having a disease with no cure.

Degenerative Disorders

Degenerative disorders are diseases in which nerve cells degenerate and die. One such disorder is Parkinson's disease, in which certain nerve centers in the brain deteriorate. The characteristic symptom of Parkinson's disease is an involuntary tremor of the hands, head, or both. Between one third and one half of people with Parkinson's disease develop depression. Most researchers think depression is a component of Parkinson's disease rather than a psychological reaction to it.

Huntington's chorea is a very rare, hereditary, degenerative nerve disease that starts in middle age. Uncontrollable body movements gradually develop over time and are followed by mental deterioration. Depression, euphoria, or other mental changes sometimes mark the early stages of Huntington's chorea.

Depression often accompanies dementia, a disorder of the brain in which there is a progressive loss of memory and other intellectual functions. People with dementia may gradually become confused, incapable of sensible conversation, and unaware of their surroundings. In Alzheimer's disease, which is responsible for most cases of dementia, depressive illness develops in up to 87 percent of people. Depression, paranoia, or delusions may accompany or result from the disease, but they can often be alleviated by appropriate treatments.

Older people may experience a depression so severe that they develop problems with thinking. Depression may be mistaken for early signs of Alzheimer's disease in these instances. Unlike Alzheimer's, however, this depression is treatable. A psychologist, psychiatrist, or a neurologist can tell whether you or your loved one have Alzheimer's disease or depression.

Mania or depression may also be an early sign of multiple sclerosis. In multiple sclerosis, your nerves lose the sheaths of myelin (a fatty substance) that protect and insulate them. Symptoms vary widely, but early on, they often include passing visual problems, temporary tingling or weakness of an arm, and bladder problems. Depression, euphoria, and other mental changes may appear years before multiple sclerosis is diagnosed. These mood changes often come and go as the disease progresses.

Diseases of the Cardiovascular System

The cardiovascular system comprises the heart and blood vessels. Physical illnesses and disorders of this system can cause depression. Among people who experience a heart attack, 15 percent to 20 percent will develop clinical depression afterward. Stroke, which occurs when a rupture or blockage of a blood vessel causes injury to the brain, is a significant cause of depression. Stroke leads to depression in about half of all people hospitalized with the disorder. Symptoms of depression in stroke patients may be a result of changes in or damage to the brain caused by the stroke or a reaction to the physical side effects and limitations caused by the stroke, such as paralysis. Psychological and neurological testing may be needed to address the cause of the depression. If you experience depression after a stroke, your doctor will probably recommend both antidepressant medication and some form of counseling or psychotherapy.

Chronic Fatigue Syndrome

Chronic fatigue syndrome (CFS) is a set of symptoms that vary from person to person, but its primary signs are total exhaustion that cannot be relieved by sleep and flulike symptoms. Other symptoms include joint and muscle weakness and pain, swollen glands and recurrent sore throat, headaches, forgetfulness, and confusion. The syndrome primarily occurs in women between ages 25 and 45. CFS can strike suddenly and last for months or years. The cause may be physical; researchers have found links between CFS and several viruses. Other researchers think that it may be a form of depressive illness, since many people with CFS experience changes in mood. Some researchers think it is a combination of both. Many researchers and physicians believe that how well the immune system is functioning is a key factor. A diagnosis of CFS requires that major clinical depression be ruled out as the primary diagnosis.

Diseases of Metabolism

The process by which your body converts food and oxygen into energy may lead to symptoms of depression. Acute intermittent porphyria is one of a group of very rare diseases caused by an inherited defect in the enzymes that produce a constituent of blood. The disease attacks the nervous system, and symptoms can include nausea, vomiting, constipation, muscle weakness, vision problems, paralysis, and mental changes. Depression is common in acute intermittent porphyria, especially between attacks.

Wilson's disease is a very rare inherited disorder in which there is an abnormal accumulation of copper in the body, particularly in the liver, cornea, and brain. Mania and depression can be among the early symptoms of this disease.

Other Physical Causes

VITAMIN DEFICIENCIES

Serious and prolonged vitamin deficiencies can bring on depression in some people. Depression is among the symptoms of pellagra, a disease caused by a lack of niacin and other B-complex vitamins in the diet. Depression and other mental changes can also be early signs that your body lacks adequate amounts of vitamin B_{12}. If untreated, vitamin B_{12} deficiency leads to a disease called pernicious anemia, which can cause a severe depletion of red blood cells in your body. Depression can also be a sign that your body is lacking folic acid, vitamin B_6 (pyridoxine), or vitamin B_1 (thiamin).

MINERAL DEFICIENCIES

Too few minerals may also cause depression. Depression can be an early symptom of iron deficiency and may accompany the disease that comes from this deficiency, called anemia. Depression may also be caused by a shortage in your body's supply of sodium, magnesium, or zinc. By contrast, an excessive amount of calcium in the blood can give rise to depression.

POISONING

Poisoning by certain substances may also bring on depressive illness. For example, adults whose bodies absorb lead often show symptoms of depression, and workers in manganese mines have been known to become manic from regularly inhaling dust from the metal manganese. Mercury poisoning can cause severe depression. Long-term exposure to low levels of arsenic—an ingredient in insecticides, herbicides, and rat poisons—can lead to depression. Poisoning by bismuth, an ingredient in skin-lightening creams and some laxatives, can cause depression that comes and goes. Large doses of bromides, substances that in the past were widely used as sedative and anticonvulsant medication, can also cause depression. Depression results from aluminum poisoning, which generally affects only people who receive kidney dialysis, the method by which waste products are removed from the blood of people with diseased kidneys through a machine that acts as an artificial kidney. In one study, 86 percent of the people receiving dialysis developed symptoms of major depression.

WHEN SUBSTANCE ABUSE CAUSES DEPRESSION

Substance abuse, a problem that occurs among all age groups, is closely linked to depression. Substance abuse is the continued use of alcohol or another substance even when it causes problems in one's life. Severe substance abuse causes physical and psychological dependence on the substance. Abused substances include alcohol, cocaine, amphetamines, heroin, some prescription medications, and other substances. All of these substances can cause depression. This link with depression may seem surprising, because people try to use alcohol and drugs to improve their mood. But taking such substances helps to cheer them up only temporarily. In the meantime, drugs of abuse may alter brain chemistry so that depressive illness can take hold.

The relationship between substance abuse and depressive illness is not always clear-cut. Take alcoholism as an example. Alcoholism is a form of drug abuse characterized by an overwhelming need for—or dependency on—alcohol. Some people who suffer from alcoholism develop depression as a result of their drinking. Other people are already depressed to begin with and drink heavily to help themselves feel better.

Drugs and alcohol cause or aggravate depressive illness by interacting with the body's mood regulator, the limbic system. When you do something that makes you feel good, such as eating a tasty meal, it is your limbic system that produces in your body a feeling of pleasure. Your pleasure response is the reward for eating, an action your brain knows is essential for survival.

Addictive substances also activate your limbic system. They do this by flooding your brain with certain neurotransmitters that make you feel good. Cocaine, for example, triggers the release of the neurotransmitter dopamine, which produces a feeling of well-being. Repeated cocaine use makes your brain release excessive amounts of dopamine. Because cocaine interferes with how nerve cells reabsorb dopamine, it ultimately depletes your brain's store of dopamine. Other brain changes can occur with the abuse of many addictive substances. These changes may either bring on depression or worsen depression that already exists.

As a result, drug dependency, including alcoholism, and depressive illness are closely connected. About half of people with alcoholism are also clinically depressed. Heavy drinkers have significantly higher rates of suicide than do other people, and suicide is closely linked with clinical depression. As many as 80 percent of cocaine abusers feel depressed at some point in their illness. At the same time, about 25 percent of people with major depression have a diagnosable substance abuse problem.

If your depression is caused by substance abuse, you and your doctor will probably decide whether to treat the substance abuse first or at the same time as your depression. As your body becomes free of the addictive substance and you confront your addiction through counseling or a 12-step program, the depression may lift by itself. This is likely to happen in cases in which the depression was produced by the drug abuse. If your depression lingers after your substance abuse is treated, however, your doctor will probably treat your depression as a separate disorder.

PRESCRIPTION MEDICATION AND DEPRESSION

Some prescription medication can cause depression. Those most likely to develop depression as a result of prescription medication include people who are genetically prone to depressive illness because it runs in their family and those who have already had an episode of depression. Also at risk are older people, whose bodies respond differently to medication.

Note that when the source of the illness is medication, the depression generally begins within days or weeks of starting the medication. Often, doctors will treat the depression simply by discontinuing the medication. In some cases, your depression may linger after the medication is changed. If so, your doctor will probably treat the depression as a separate disorder.

Research shows that more than 200 medications have caused depression in certain individuals, but doctors know of only a few medications that frequently cause depression, including certain ones for high blood pressure and Parkinson's disease. Medications for high blood pressure, such as reserpine, methyldopa, guanethidine, propranolol, and clonidine, are suspected of causing significant depression in some people. Reserpine and methyldopa seem particularly likely to do so. At least 15 percent of people who take reserpine develop depressive illness, though many of these people had a history of depression.

Drugs used to treat Parkinson's disease include L-dopa, which causes mental changes in about 1 of 5 people who use it. These mental changes can include depression and mild mania.

Among other prescription medications linked to depression are certain nonsteroidal anti-inflammatory drugs (NSAIDs), corticosteroid medications, anabolic steroids, oral contraceptives, anticonvulsant medicines, and medicine to lower cholesterol. NSAIDs are prescribed to relieve pain in osteoarthritis, rheumatoid arthritis, and other joint diseases. Anticonvulsant medications, which are used to treat seizures, may also lead to depression. One such anticonvulsant, phenobarbital, is particularly likely to bring on depression, especially in people who have a family or personal history of the mood disorder.

Corticosteroid medications are used to treat Addison's disease, allergies, rheumatic disorders, and inflammation. Mental changes, including depression, occur in about 5 percent of the people who use these medications.

Oral contraceptives, which contain the sex hormones estrogen and progesterone, are used to prevent pregnancy. The connection between oral contraceptives and depression is controversial. Most research has found that oral contraceptives may cause depression, but some studies have contradicted this. In general, researchers believe that women who have previously had depression may be at the highest risk for developing it while using oral contraceptives.

Anabolic steroids can cause depression in some people. Anabolic steroids are sometimes prescribed to treat certain kinds of anemia and advanced breast cancer. Some athletes use or abuse them to improve muscle strength and endurance, though such use is unwise and illegal in competitive sports.

Some studies have suggested that medication to lower your blood cholesterol level may bring on depression, though other studies have refuted this theory. Cholesterol is a fatty substance found in some foods. High amounts of cholesterol in the blood have been linked to heart disease.

INTERRELATED CAUSES

The causes of depression may be interrelated. Some researchers think depressive illness is actually a number of different disorders, each caused by a different problem. According to this theory, flaws in the biological clock cause some cases of depressive illness, while others are caused by abnormal brain chemistry, and still others are caused by stressful situations. Other researchers think most depressive illness is caused by several factors that work together to make you ill, such as unusual stress combined with a genetic vulnerability. There are also many unknowns surrounding depression. Researchers still do not know, for example, why depressive illness hits only some people with a genetic predisposition and not others. Despite all the uncertainty, doctors note that our understanding of depressive illness is advancing rapidly. In another generation, we may completely understand what brings about depressive illness—and why.

5

Getting Help for Depression

If you have depressive illness, you may think that nobody can understand how you feel or that nothing can help you feel better. In fact, this hopeless feeling is often a symptom of depression. Other people can understand you and help you. Depressive illness is one of the most treatable mental illnesses. About 80 percent of depressed people experience significant improvement with professional help, often within weeks or months.

DO I NEED HELP?

Sometimes it is hard to admit you need a doctor's help. You may equate depression with other forms of mental illness, such as schizophrenia. Or you may see your symptoms as a weakness or character flaw. Perhaps you fear your friends, family, or boss will be uncomfortable with you once they know you are depressed. Despite advances in understanding the causes of depressive illness, it still carries a stigma to many people.

It always hurts to acknowledge that you are ill, because doing so changes your idea of yourself. It is especially hard to accept an illness that affects your mind, since the mind is often regarded as the center or seat of the self.

In addition, your symptoms may prevent you from seeking help. The fatigue of depressive illness can make going to the doctor seem overwhelming. Your illness may also prompt you to withdraw from others and conceal the severity of your symptoms. If you are in the manic phase of bipolar depression, you probably lack the insight to realize that you are ill.

Before you admit you need help, you may go through several emotional stages. At first, you may be in pain without knowing you are depressed. You may be unable to put your feelings into words. If you have been depressed for a long time, despondency may seem part of your personality. You can probably find an excuse for why you are sad—a relationship that went wrong, a missed promotion, or a fight with a neighbor. Later, you may slowly sense that something is amiss. By then, your pain may make everyday life a struggle. Finally, you seek professional help. Like many people, you may need a crisis, such as losing a job, to become convinced that you can no longer ignore your suffering.

Do you wonder whether you have depressive illness? If so, read the checklist on the next page and mark the symptoms that apply to you. It may help to ask your spouse or a close friend if any of these symptoms appear to belong to you.

CHECKLIST FOR DEPRESSION

- Feeling sad, anxious, or empty, always or most of the time
- Thinking about death or suicide
- Feeling guilty, hopeless, or worthless
- Losing interest or pleasure in activities that used to be fun, including sex
- Sleeping too little or too much
- Eating less than usual and losing weight without dieting, or eating more than usual and gaining weight
- Being restless or irritable
- Experiencing persistent physical ailments that never respond to treatment, such as headaches, chronic pain, or constipation and other digestive problems
- Finding it hard to concentrate, remember things, or make up your mind
- Running low on energy

If you checked four to five or more symptoms, including the first two, and if these symptoms have persisted for more than 2 weeks, you may have depressive illness. Now is the time to discuss these feelings with a doctor. Even if you have only some of these symptoms, talk about them with your doctor. A few symptoms now can deepen into major depression later. You may already have a mild form of depression.

Perhaps you have symptoms of depression but think your feelings are healthy. For example, if you are getting divorced and do not have enough money to pay your bills, it is natural to worry or feel bad. How can you tell if your feelings are symptoms that need treatment? One way is to look at how well you can meet your various obligations. Can you put in a good day's work? Do you see your friends and family members and have a good time in their company? Are you at ease in social situations? If you are often unhappy but can live your normal life, you probably are not clinically depressed. On the other hand, you may do well in one area of your life but not in others because you are depressed. Some depressed people do just fine at work, for example, but withdraw socially. If you cannot cope with some aspects of your life, you probably should talk to your doctor.

If you have bipolar depression, the symptoms on the depression checklist will apply to you only at certain times. At other times, you will experience mania, or extreme joy, and your symptoms will be entirely different. If you are manic right now, you are highly unlikely to suspect anything is wrong. But if your mania has passed, some of its symptoms might sound familiar. Look at the checklist below and mark any symptoms that apply to you. It may help to ask a close friend or family member if they have noticed symptoms in you.

CHECKLIST FOR MANIA

- Feeling unusually happy, euphoric, or irritable
- Being able to go several days without sleep
- Talking a great deal or being unable to stop talking
- Being easily distracted
- Thinking up many ideas very quickly and simultaneously
- Doing things that feel good but that have undesirable consequences, such as spending too much money or engaging in sexual behavior that is unusual for you
- Feeling that you are vastly important to others
- Planning many projects or major changes in your life or feeling that you have to keep moving

Having several of these symptoms at once for at least 1 week, including the first symptom, may point to mania. If this sounds like you, tell your doctor.

DOES SOMEONE YOU LOVE NEED HELP?

Some people cannot see how ill they are. They need to be encouraged to seek treatment by friends or family. Maybe you care for somebody who may have a depressive illness. Look at the two checklists and answer the questions. If the person you care for meets the criteria as described, he or she needs help.

Convincing someone to seek help for depressive illness can be difficult, especially if he or she has mania. Suppose you think your sister has depressive illness. How can you get her to take you seriously? There is no sure way to do so, but try sharing your impression that something is seriously wrong. Tell her why you are worried. Mention changes you have noticed in her thinking, physical well-being, or behavior. Tell her you want to help her tackle the problem, whatever it turns out to be. Try to maintain a supportive tone in the conversation, rather than an argumentative tone. Stress that it is not that you are trying to pass her problems on to someone else but that you just want a doctor to be a partner in solving the problem.

Try to avoid framing her problem in an overly technical or pessimistic way. Avoid the phrase "mental illness" because of the negative connotations of those words. Point out that her symptoms may be caused by an unrecognized medical problem. Urge her to see an expert who can pinpoint what is wrong. If she resists the idea, ask her to see a doctor just to humor you. Suggest visiting the doctor together. If your sister agrees that something is wrong, she would probably like some reassurance.

Sometimes it is too hard to initiate a conversation about getting help, and you may need to wait for an opening provided by the other person. For example, your sister may say, "I just don't know what to do about my daughter's problems." Then you can take the opportunity to say that it could be helpful to talk to a professional.

Whenever you suspect someone is depressed, find out if he or she is suicidal. Do not be evasive. Ask straight out: "Have you felt that life isn't worth living? Are you thinking about killing yourself?" Many people, including some doctors, are wary of asking such a blunt question. Asking the question will not plant the idea of suicide in the depressed person's mind. In fact, if you discuss the possibility of suicide, the other person is less likely to kill himself or herself. Simply by raising the topic, you lessen the other person's isolation and defuse the situation. He or she may be relieved to talk about these frightening thoughts. If your loved one admits to feeling suicidal, get medical help immediately.

For more information on helping your loved one with depression, see Chapter 7.

HOW TREATMENT CAN HELP

Many depressed people avoid seeking treatment. If you are depressed, you may doubt that any treatment can be helpful. If your depression is recurring, perhaps you have managed to get through bouts of your illness before without treatment and emerged feeling better. Medical treatment can, however, make your pain go away faster. Most people who receive the correct treatment feel well enough to resume their normal activities after several weeks. Left untreated, depressive illness does usually get better, but it can take a long time to do so.

Maybe you think you should be able to snap out of your blue

mood without anyone's help. What you are feeling, though, may be depressive illness rather than a blue mood, and depressive illness is not as easily shaken. After all, if you could banish your depression through an act of will, you would have done it by now.

The sooner you seek help, the more likely you are to recover. As with any illness, depression becomes entrenched and more difficult to treat over time. Early treatment greatly increases your chance of a full recovery. And the benefits you receive while you get treatment, discussed below, are well worth the effort.

Saving a Life

Seeking help can save your life. People who have a depressive illness, especially an untreated one, are much more likely than people who are healthy to commit suicide. Most people who act suicidal do so because of untreated mental illness, substance abuse, or both. If you had another potentially fatal disease, such as breast cancer, you probably would rush to get treatment. Why should depressive illness be any different?

Helping a Relationship

Tackling your illness may help important relationships survive. Your illness has probably put great strain on your marriage or partnership, friendships, and family ties. Many symptoms, from the social withdrawal of depression to the heightened sexuality of mania, foster conflict and misunderstanding. Marriages are particularly hard hit. If you are depressed, your marriage is nine times more likely to end in divorce than a marriage between two healthy people. About 50 percent of depressed women say they have serious marital difficulties. Depressive illness, and the sexual problems it causes, is one of the most common reasons couples seek counseling. If you get treatment now, you can stop the damage and start the healing.

Improving Your Physical Health

Treating your depression will boost not only your mental health but also your physical health. Depressive illness leeches your power to rebound from physical injuries. Experts say, for example, that if you suffer a hip fracture while depressed, your recovery will take longer than that of a healthy person. People with depression are also more likely to smoke. Smoking increases your risk of heart disease, lung disease, certain cancers, and many other ailments. And if you have a serious medical illness and a depressive illness, depression decreases your chances of getting well.

Nobody is sure why depression negatively affects people's chances of recovery in this way. Some researchers believe that depression can reduce the effectiveness of your immune system, which defends you against disease. Another theory is that depression makes seriously ill people less likely to follow doctor's orders or take medication as prescribed.

Helping You Avoid Impulsive Actions

If you have bipolar depression, seeking treatment can shield you from the pain and embarrassment that can result from manic behavior. Many people emerge from mania to find they are in some kind of trouble, such as deep debt, as a result of their mania. The consequences of manic behavior can be long-lasting and painful. Treatment can help ensure that you never have to face such consequences again.

WHERE TO FIND HELP

The first step toward finding help for your depression is to have your illness properly diagnosed. Only then can you decide who will treat you and where. If you have a family doctor, you should probably turn to him or her first for a diagnosis.

If you do not have a regular doctor, contact your local medical society, community mental health clinic, health department, or hospital and explain your situation. Many schools have counselors on staff who can make referrals. Some employers provide mental health counseling through employee assistance programs, which can also help with referrals. Or ask friends, family, or a religious advisor to recommend a good doctor. If this research seems too exhausting or difficult to contemplate, try asking your spouse, a family member, or a friend to make a few calls on your behalf.

Check with your employer or insurance company to see what sorts of treatment for mental health are covered under your policy. Many insurance policies do not fully cover costs for treating mental illness, so you may want to ask your doctor about available options.

GETTING A DIAGNOSIS

No simple test can tell whether you have depression. To a large extent, your doctor will base the diagnosis on what you say about your symptoms, your general health, your medical history, and your family's history of physical and mental illnesses. The more forthcoming you are, the more accurate your diagnosis will be. In addition, your doctor will give you a physical examination, perform laboratory tests to make sure your depression is not caused by physical illness (see Chapter 4), and possibly will run additional tests to confirm the diagnosis.

What to Tell the Doctor

Your doctor will check for signs of depression by questioning you about your mood, behavior, and physical well-being. You probably will discuss how well you have been sleeping, whether you have been confused or indecisive lately, and whether you have been unusually sad or happy. It may help to bring the checklist of symptoms from earlier in this chapter. Your doctor will ask how long you have been feeling this way, what makes your symptoms better or worse, and whether you have tried to relieve your symptoms with medication.

Because depressive illness distorts your thinking, answering your doctor's questions may not be easy. For example, if you are severely depressed, you may find it impossible to answer the doctor's questions with more than a few words. If you are manic or hypomanic, you may lack the judgment to describe your symptoms. You may find it helpful to bring a close friend or family member along to provide additional background information as well as an objective description of your recent actions.

Your doctor will ask you detailed questions about your health history, past and present. A stroke or a recent bout of mononucleosis, for example, could explain your symptoms of depression. Your doctor will also ask about past treatments and medications.

Your doctor will use this information to help determine the possible causes of your depression and to devise effective treatment, so make sure the history you give is complete. If you are depressed right now, for example, but fail to tell your doctor that you had hypomania in the past, he or she may prescribe a medication that could tip you into mania.

Again, your symptoms may cloud your ability to be accurate. For example, if you are deeply depressed, you may tell your doctor that a certain antidepressant was totally ineffective in the past. In fact, the antidepressant may have helped, but your memory is now somewhat distorted by the depression. Information about medication is particularly important because many doctors prefer to prescribe an antidepressant that has already worked for you. A close friend or family member who knows your medical history may help clarify matters.

Some of your doctor's questions may be personal. He or she may ask you about your interest in sex, for example, or about your use of drugs or alcohol. You may feel embarrassed about answering, but everything you tell your doctor is confidential. It is important to answer these questions as honestly as you can because everything you say can affect your diagnosis and treatment. Your description of your drinking habits, for example, may help your doctor decide a course of treatment. Alcohol abuse can cause or aggravate depression. If your doctor knows you drink heavily, he or she may decide to treat you for substance abuse first and see if this makes the depression go away.

Your doctor will want to know about your family's health, especially whether any of your relatives have or have had mental illness. This fact could be significant, since mood disorders tend to run in families. Any details you can offer about the treatment of your relative's mental illness may be useful. For example, an antidepressant that helped your father, may also work for you—or it may not. The more details you can provide, the better.

Giving Your Health History

It may be easier to answer your doctor's questions if you prepare for them ahead of time. Answering these questions before your doctor's visit, perhaps with the help of a spouse or friend, may help your visit go more smoothly:

1. Do you have a physical illness now—for example, cancer, arthritis, or diseases that affect your heart, thyroid, or nervous system? What physical illnesses have you had? When did you have them and for how long? How were they treated?

2. Have you ever had episodes of depression, hypomania, or mania? When and for how long? How were they treated?

3. Do you have a mental illness now? Have you had a mental illness in the past? When and for how long? How was it treated?

4. What drugs, including alcohol, do you use? How often do you use them and in what amounts?

5. What medications, prescription or over the counter, do you take regularly? Include everything, from the cold capsules you use every winter to the pain reliever you take every month when your period arrives.

6. Are you allergic to food, medication, or anything else? What is your reaction? How do you treat this allergy?

7. Do any illnesses run in your family, such as diabetes, thy-

roid disease, heart disease, depression, or substance abuse? Mention any relative who has or has had a depressive illness, another mental illness (especially if he or she was hospitalized), or a substance abuse problem. Mention any relative who has committed or attempted suicide, who has a nervous system disease such as Parkinson's disease, or who has an unknown illness.

8. What recent changes or stresses have you had? Include positive changes, such as a promotion at work or a move to a bigger house.
9. What additional information may be helpful?

Answering your doctor's questions is important, but so is volunteering information. If anything comes to mind, mention it. What you may think is unimportant or be tempted to leave out may turn out to be very helpful.

Physical Examination and Laboratory Tests

To make sure your depression is not due to a physical illness, your doctor will give you a complete physical examination. Between 10 percent and 15 percent of cases of depressive illness are caused by medical conditions. In addition, your doctor may order blood tests and a urine test to check for abnormal levels of certain hormones, including thyroid and cortisol, nutritional deficiencies, and other factors. These tests are performed in order to rule out chronic medical problems that can cause symptoms of depression, including diabetes, disorders of the thyroid and adrenal glands, and kidney and liver abnormalities (see Chapter 4).

The tests you receive may vary with your age and medical

history. Depression in a person with several risk factors is less likely to be caused by physical illness than depression in a person with few risk factors. Suppose you are a 70-year-old man who is depressed for the first time and no one in your family has ever had depressive illness. Your doctor will first look for one of the many physical illnesses that causes depression, since it is unusual for depression to strike for the first time at your age. On the other hand, suppose that you are a 20-year-old woman with several family members who have had depressive illness, and you have already experienced two bouts of major depression. You will probably receive fewer tests than the older person—maybe only routine checks for thyroid disease, nutritional deficiencies, or mononucleosis—because your medical history points to a return episode of major depression.

Three additional, more sophisticated clinical tests are some-times used to identify certain hormonal, brain, or sleep abnormal-ities linked to depression. They are used mainly in research and academic settings, such as teaching hospitals, and are more likely to be used if your depression is severe and prolonged. A negative result on the tests does not rule out depression. Since you may still have depression even if the tests fail to find abnormalities, these tests are not used for routine screening and diagnosis. They can, however, help to confirm a diagnosis of depression and give your doctor clues about how to treat your illness. Occasionally, they can identify or suggest the presence of depression in some-one who has unusual or untypical symptoms.

DEXAMETHASONE SUPPRESSION TEST

In the dexamethasone suppression test (DST), you are given a dose of synthetic cortisol, or dexamethasone, before you go to sleep at night. The next day, your blood is tested for cortisol at 8 A.M. and 4 P.M. If you are healthy, your cortisol levels will first drop and then gradually return to normal as your hypothalamus reacts to the synthetic cortisol in your blood. In severely depressed people, about half will show an abnormal response in which cortisol levels are not suppressed or do not change after a dose of dexamethasone.

However, if you had an abnormal DST result when depressed, despite healthy adrenal glands, you may show a normal DST result when your depression subsides. Your doctor may repeat the test to confirm your depression is improving or has resolved.

THYROID-RELEASING HORMONE STIMULATION TEST

The thyroid-releasing hormone (TRH) stimulation test shows whether your body's system for secreting thyroid hormone, which involves a series of signals from your brain to your pituitary gland to your thyroid, is working normally. This system is abnormal in about 30 percent to 60 percent of severely depressed people.

First, a blood sample will be drawn to measure your normal levels of thyroid-stimulating hormone (TSH), the hormone that sends the thyroid into action. Then, you will receive a dose of TRH, the hormone that controls TSH production. Your blood TSH level will be measured again 15, 30, and 90 minutes later. If your thyroid is healthy, blood samples will show your levels of TSH have risen.

RAPID EYE MOVEMENT LATENCY

Rapid eye movement (REM) latency is the length of time between the start of sleep and the beginning of REM sleep. These sleep cycles are abnormal in 40 percent to 60 percent of clinically depressed people (see Chapter 3). Your doctor may order a test that measures your sleep cycles. Measurements are made through a device called an electroencephalograph (EEG), which produces a recording called an electroencephalogram that detects the electrical activity of the brain painlessly through the skin. The test usually takes place overnight in a hospital equipped with a sleep laboratory. During the test, skin electrodes are attached to your scalp. The electrodes conduct the brain's electrical waves to the EEG, which records them. An electroencephalogram, or recording of the brain's activity, is then made while you sleep. This recording can tell the doctor whether your sleep is normal. If your sleep is abnormal, it may give your doctor clues about which form of treatment will be best for you.

QUESTIONING YOUR DIAGNOSIS

Your symptoms, your medical and family history, and your test results all help your doctor diagnose your illness. You may accept this diagnosis or question it. Sometimes the nature of your illness makes you reject the diagnosis even when it is correct. People with bipolar depression, for instance, rarely accept their first diagnosis. This inability to acknowledge the illness is sometimes called denial.

In other cases, your doctor's diagnosis may be incorrect. Depressive illness is often overlooked or confused with something else. Two thirds of people with depressive illness never learn they have it. Researchers have found that doctors do not diagnose depression in about 50 percent of the depressed people who see them. Doctors are especially unlikely to spot the kinds of depression that are marked by such physical complaints as insomnia and fatigue but no sadness. In addition, your doctor's diagnosis may be biased. Researchers have found, for example, that a doctor is more likely to diagnose your bipolar depression as schizophrenia if you belong to a different ethnic group than your doctor.

If you think your doctor's diagnosis is wrong—or simply want to make sure it is correct—ask for a referral to another doctor for a second opinion. Many people seek a second opinion when they feel uncomfortable about their doctor's diagnosis. Asking for one will not strain your relationship with your doctor.

SELECTING TREATMENT

Once you are certain that you have depressive illness, you and your doctor must decide how to treat it. Treatment options for depression include medication, psychotherapy (talk therapy), electroconvulsive therapy (ECT), and light therapy. Your choice of treatment will depend on the form of depressive illness, its severity, the cost of treatment, and your preference for treatment.

People with bipolar depression usually need to remain on medication to control the symptoms. Psychotherapy can help people accept that their bipolar depression will require lifelong medication.

Some doctors think psychotherapy by itself is the best treatment for mild to moderate depression. You have mild depression when you have some symptoms of depression and must push yourself to carry out your day-to-day activities. You have moderate depression when you have many symptoms that often prevent you from doing the things you need to do.

People with major depression have more options. You have

major depression when you have nearly all the symptoms and they almost always keep you from leading your normal life. For moderate to severe major depression, your doctor will probably recommend medication or a combination of medication and psychotherapy. For a thorough discussion of treatments for depression, see Chapter 6.

Selecting a treatment often comes to weighing its pros and cons. For example, your doctor may recommend a particular medication that is likely to provide relief (pro) but may also bring negative side effects (con) or be very expensive (con). When you discuss possible treatments with your doctor, have a list of questions ready. You may want to ask questions like these:

- How likely am I to get better with this treatment?
- How soon will I feel better?
- Will this treatment make me entirely well or just improve my condition?
- What side effects and risks does this treatment entail?
- What are the costs of this treatment?
- How will this treatment affect my lifestyle?
- What are other treatment alternatives?

Your doctor's answers will help you make the right choice.

WHO TREATS DEPRESSIVE ILLNESS?

Several different kinds of practitioners treat depressive illness, which can be confusing. You may end up seeing more than one, depending on the type of treatment that is right for you. Some conditions, such as severe major depression or bipolar depression, require medication. Any licensed physician, such as your family doctor or a psychiatrist, can write prescriptions. Psychologists, social workers, and counselors can provide psychotherapy but cannot prescribe medication. A person who provides psychotherapy is often called a psychotherapist or therapist, regardless of his or her profession. Which professional(s) you work with depend on many factors: how severe your illness is, who is available in your area, whether your health insurance covers specialized care, or how much you can afford to pay for treatment.

Family doctors, physician assistants, nurse practitioners, and other health-care providers treat depressive illness and other medical problems but do not specialize in treating mental illness. Sometimes you or your doctor may think it best that you see a mental health specialist. Your doctor may suggest a specialist if you have a severe form of depressive illness, such as bipolar depression; if your depression persists despite treatment; or if you need certain treatments such as psychotherapy, ECT, or light therapy. In many cases, you will continue to see your doctor as well as the specialist. For example, you might see your doctor for medication and a social worker for psychotherapy. Mental health specialists include psychiatrists, psychologists, social workers, and psychiatric nurses.

Family Doctor

A family doctor diagnoses and treats most health problems for people of all ages, from a newborn's nursing blister to a grandmother's high blood pressure. He or she has some training in treating mental illness but does not specialize in it. The doctor's qualifications include a 4-year bachelor's degree, a 4-year medical degree, and at least 3 years' training in a hospital under the supervision of experienced doctors. In addition, your doctor is licensed by the state, which requires passing an examination. Even when your family doctor refers you to a specialist, he or she often remains in charge of overseeing or coordinating your treatment.

You may be happy to have your family doctor treat your depression. After all, this is a person you already know and probably like and trust. He or she already knows your medical history and is used to dealing with your health problems. About half of people with mental illness are treated by their family doctor or internist, a doctor who specializes in diagnosing and treating diseases of adults. In addition, most prescriptions for antidepressants are written by family doctors. (Many people feel less embarrassed about seeking help from their regular doctor than from a specialist in mental health.) In general, your family doctor or internist can handle milder cases of major depression. Also, some health insurance providers may be more likely to reimburse the cost of treatment if it is provided by the family doctor.

Physician's Assistant and Nurse Practitioner

Other health-care providers may help with your treatment, often working in the same office as your doctor. For example, you may receive some routine care from a physician's assistant, a person with medical knowledge and some training in mental illness. A physician's assistant is not a doctor but is certified to work under your doctor's supervision. Or you may see a nurse practitioner, a professional nurse with additional training, including some in treating mental illness. Today, nurse practitioners do a lot of work previously reserved for doctors. They are registered nurses (RNs) who have a 4-year or 5-year bachelor of science degree or an approved 3-year diploma. In addition, RNs are licensed, which entails passing a special examination.

Psychiatrist

A psychiatrist is a medical doctor who specializes in diagnosing and treating mental illness. Your psychiatrist can give you several kinds of care. He or she can prescribe antidepressant medication, provide psychotherapy, or both. In addition, only a psychiatrist can perform ECT. A psychiatrist has a 4-year bachelor's degree, a 4-year medical degree, and at least 4 years of training in mental illness as a resident in a hospital. A psychiatrist is fully qualified to diagnose and differentiate physical illness from mental illness. You will probably see a psychiatrist if your depressive illness is severe—for example, if you are suicidal or have lost touch with reality.

Psychologist

A psychologist is an expert in how the mind works. Psychologists seek to understand why you act, think, and feel as you do. They are not able to prescribe medication, but they do provide psychological testing and psychotherapy. Those who specialize in mental illness are called clinical psychologists. Although you may call your clinical psychologist "doctor," this title refers to a doctoral degree, which usually requires 2 or 3 additional years of study beyond a master's degree. In addition, clinical psychologists work for at least 1 year as an intern under the supervision of experienced therapists, and they write a dissertation on a research topic.

Psychologists are licensed by the state, which requires passing a special examination.

Psychiatric Nurse

A psychiatric nurse is a registered nurse who specializes in treating mental illness. He or she may dispense medication ordered by your psychiatrist or check you for side effects. Some psychiatric nurses are trained to provide psychotherapy. Most have a master's degree in addition to their nurse's training.

Social Worker

A social worker is trained to help you deal with personal problems. You may see a social worker for psychotherapy, alone or in a group; for training in the skills of everyday living; or during a crisis. Your social worker can advise you on many problems, from claiming disability payments to telling your children about your illness. Most social workers who specialize in mental health have a master's degree and specialized training in counseling.

Other Assistance

Health professionals are not the only people who can help you cope with depressive illness. Many depressed people first seek help from their priest, minister, or rabbi. In fact, of all people who seek counseling for their problems, about 40 percent consult a member of the clergy before going to see a doctor, psychologist, or social worker. In addition, your religious advisor may notice your depression before anyone else and may make it a point to speak to you about it.

Members of the clergy may not be able personally to help you deal with depressive illness, but they can comfort you and reassure you that you are right to seek help, and they may be able to refer you to a psychiatrist or psychologist. Some clergy members have special training in counseling; they are often called pastoral counselors. Your pastoral counselor will work closely with your physician or psychiatrist and may consult with your religious advisor.

A support group, made up of other people who share problems similar to yours, may also help you accept and learn more about your illness. It will probably be a relief to discuss your illness with people who have had similar experiences. You may have questions that you are embarrassed to raise with your doctor but can more easily ask of your support group. Group members can help you realize that having an illness does not make you a damaged person. A support group is no substitute for professional care, but it can help you learn to live with your illness.

CHOOSING YOUR PROFESSIONAL CARE

Regardless of who treats you, you will want to look for certain qualities in that person. Your practitioner should be someone who has diagnosed and treated depressive illness before. He or she should be familiar with all the available treatments, from the many medications to the different kinds of psychotherapy. He or she should be able to explain clearly depressive illness and what is known about its causes. In addition, he or she should be straightforward about what you can and cannot expect from treatment. You will appreciate having a doctor or therapist who can empathize as you go through depression, mania, or hypomania. The personal and professional connection between the two of you can be a steady source of comfort.

You may prefer a practitioner who sees you as a partner in your treatment. Signs of this attitude include talking to you as an intelligent equal, welcoming your questions, and being willing to change tactics if your treatment does not work. Whenever possible, your practitioner should include you in the process of making decisions about your treatment. He or she should be willing and able to see you frequently, especially at the beginning, to make sure your treatment is working. Your practitioner should accept his or her limitations and refer you to someone else when you feel it is necessary.

You also have a role in helping your treatment go well. The more you know about your illness, the better. Follow your practitioner's recommendations and keep every appointment, whether you feel ill or well. Be honest about how the treatment is working, and speak up about any concerns such as side effects of medications. Accept that it may take time to find the right treatment. Try to give yourself a few days to adjust to a new medication, rather than quickly deciding you cannot adjust to it. This may be difficult at times, especially if your illness makes you feel hopeless or apathetic. It may help to tell a family member or close friend about your treatment, so that he or she can encourage you when you feel frustrated.

If you feel that your relationship with your practitioner is not what it should be, speak up. Explain to him or her what you think is lacking. If the practitioner does not respond to your concerns, ask for a referral to somebody else. Many people with depression meet with several health-care practitioners before finding one with whom they are fully satisfied.

WHERE WILL I BE TREATED?

The place where you receive treatment typically depends on who treats you. Most people with depression get their treatment through regular visits to a doctor, therapist, or both. Some practitioners have private offices, while others work in hospitals or community mental health clinics.

In some parts of the country, clinics that specialize in research on and treatment of depressive illness are part of a university's department of psychiatry or psychology. You can call these departments for more information. Such clinics can offer advanced care, particularly for complicated situations.

Other areas have teaching clinics, which are also affiliated with universities. You can get more information by calling the university's department of psychiatry or psychology. If you attend such a clinic, you may see a resident who is training under experienced doctors. One drawback of teaching clinics is that each resident works there for only a limited time. Unless your care is short term, you may find yourself working with more than one resident.

Private treatment is usually provided in an office. In general, a psychiatrist is the most expensive provider, a psychologist less expensive, and a social worker least expensive.

In some cases, you may be treated in the hospital. Hospitalization generally is necessary if you can no longer care for yourself or are dangerous to yourself or others. If you are deeply depressed, suicidal, or manic, you will need hospital care until your treatment takes hold. When depressed people are hospitalized, it is usually for only a few days up to a week or two; on rare occasions, it may be longer. Your chances of being hospitalized are lower if you seek treatment early, before your depression becomes severe.

If you have health insurance and hope to reclaim the cost of your treatment, your family doctor will probably refer you to a particular specialist. Some health insurance plans require that the specialist be selected from a certain group of health-care providers. When getting a referral, ask for several names, if possible. That way, you can pick the person you like best or the place that is most convenient.

If you do not have health insurance or if your insurance excludes mental health care, look for a community mental health clinic in your area that offers treatment based on your income and ability to pay. You can find such a clinic by checking a phone book, calling a local hospital, or talking to your minister, pastor, or rabbi. If you know somebody who has been treated for mental illness, that person might be able to steer you toward a local clinic. Public-service organizations, such as your local health department or one of the support groups listed at the end of this book, might also have information. If you go to a community mental health clinic, you will probably see a doctor only for evaluation and medication and receive psychotherapy from a social worker or a psychologist.

HELPING YOURSELF

Depression is an illness that requires medical treatment, which is discussed in the next chapter. But even as you are seeking treatment for your depression, you can do much on your own to help yourself feel better. Making some of the following changes to your daily life may hasten your recovery.

- **Be kind to yourself.** Admit that your illness saps your energy, preventing you from doing all the things you used to. Try not to set difficult goals or accept too much responsibility. Break your large tasks into smaller steps and do what you can. Avoid criticizing yourself for not achieving more. If possible, avoid making significant life changes such as switching jobs or getting married; this is not the best time. Remember that depression clouds your judgment.
- **Lessen the amount of stress in your life.** Learning to lessen stress is difficult. Try to identify the situations and behaviors that cause you the most stress and look for specific ways to avoid the situation or change the behavior. For instance, if you know that you are chronically late to work and important appointments and that this causes you considerable stress, make a conscious decision to aim for an earlier-than-needed arrival time.
- **Exercise regularly.** Thirty minutes of exercise at least 3 days a week may boost your mood within a few weeks. Exercise reduces stress, relieves muscle tension, and often lifts your spirits. Doctors think it has this effect by improving your circulation and boosting your brain's supply of oxygen. In addition, it releases chemicals called endorphins and enkephalins, which are natural antidepressants.
- **Stick to a routine.** Find a routine that suits you and stick to it as much as possible. Get up at the same time every morning,

eat at set times, and go to bed early enough to get a good night's sleep. Many people with depressive illness, particularly bipolar depression, feel worse when they get too little sleep. Following a routine may reset your biological clock, which is often disrupted during depressive illness.

• **Educate yourself.** The more you know about depression, the easier it will be to manage. Knowledge may make your illness seem less mysterious and frightening. Reading this book is a good first step in learning more about depression. Your librarian can help you locate articles, other books, and pamphlets about depression written for the lay reader. Many of the organizations listed in the Resources section at the end of this book offer free information on depression and its treatment.

• **Avoid recreational drugs and alcohol.** Illegal drugs and alcohol may help you feel better in the short run, but they will make your depression much worse over time.

• **Be aware of your thoughts.** Listen to your thoughts when you are depressed, without judging them or worrying about whether they are "correct." Do you constantly put yourself down, harp on your mistakes, or imagine catastrophe lurking? Practicing awareness of such thoughts can provide some objectivity to offset the distorted viewpoint that depression generally brings.

• **Reach out to others.** If you are depressed, you probably shun other people. But if you spend too much time alone, dwelling on your problems, you will continue to feel bad. Being with others can distract your mind from the depression. Do something you enjoy with someone else. Go to the movies, a ball game, a concert—whatever seems like potential fun. If you have loving friends or family members who understand your illness, turn to them. Many people find that support groups offer the relief of talking to people who understand.

- **Give yourself time.** Depression is a difficult illness that will not retreat overnight. Remember that recovery from depression is the rule, not the exception. Reassure yourself that recovery is on the way.

6

Treatments for Depressive Illness

Although depressive illness is treatable, no single standard treatment exists. If you have a depressive illness, your treatment will depend on the kind of illness you have and its severity. The most important thing you can do for yourself is to continue to seek help until you find a treatment that works for you so that you feel better.

In the past, many doctors were divided on the questions of how best to treat depressive illness. Some saw it as a psychological disorder to be treated mainly with psychotherapy. Others regarded it as a physical condition best treated with medication. Today, most doctors agree that both treatments have much to offer, either separately or in combination, depending on the individual and his or her symptoms.

Whatever treatment your doctor recommends, the goal is to lift your depression so that you feel better. Treatment for major depression is often in two or three steps. The first step is acute treatment, which focuses on relieving your immediate symptoms. Acute treatment usually lasts for 6 to 12 weeks. If you receive the correct acute treatment, you will feel well when it is over. The second step is continuation treatment, during which you are treated for depression even though you feel well. Continuation treatment tries to prevent a relapse and usually lasts between 4 and 9 months. If this is your first or second episode of depressive illness, you may need no more care after your continuation treatment ends.

Some people go on to the third step, which is called maintenance treatment. Maintenance treatment may last a long time, even a lifetime. It tries to prevent your depression from recurring. A relapse and a recurrence of depression are not the same thing. A relapse is a return of your current symptoms after you begin to treat them. A recurrence is a completely new episode of your illness. Generally, people who have had three or more recurrent episodes of depression receive maintenance treatment.

There is no sure cure for depressive illness, although many people never suffer more than one episode. In general, treatment aims at controlling your condition rather than curing it. Just as people with diabetes or high blood pressure learn to manage their illness, you will learn techniques to manage your illness, too.

During treatment, you will visit your doctor or therapist regularly. If you are receiving psychotherapy as treatment, you will spend visits with your therapist talking and working through various aspects of your depression. Your doctor or therapist will use these visits to make sure your symptoms are lifting, to see whether you are experiencing any side effects from medication, and to change your prescription if the medication is not working. It is important to keep your appointments, whether you are feeling better (and now believe that medication is unnecessary) or worse (and now believe medication is not helping). In some cases, you may see a therapist for psychotherapy frequently while seeing a psychiatrist periodically for medication.

Almost all treatments have potential disadvantages. Psychotherapy may take some time before you notice any change. Antidepressant medications may cause side effects that you cannot tolerate. You may have to try several treatments before anything works. Treating depression can also be expensive, especially if you lack health insurance or if the mental health benefits of your insurance are limited. But failing to treat depression is also costly—in emotional and physical pain, in time lost from work or school, in damaged relationships. Despite all the difficulties that may come with treatment, none is as difficult or as costly as the illness itself.

The most common treatments for depressive illness are medication, psychotherapy, or a combination of the two. Electroconvulsive therapy (ECT) is only for major depression; light therapy is used to treat seasonal affective disorder (SAD). Alternative therapies, such as nutritional supplements, yoga, and meditation, are sometimes used to treat depression, often to complement standard treatments.

MEDICATION

Medications are used to treat both depression and mania, especially severe major depression and bipolar depression. If you have another kind of depressive illness, you may have the option to take or not take medication. Medication helps many people, sometimes very quickly. More than 50 percent of depressed people feel significantly better or completely better after they start medication. But medication has drawbacks, too, including the expense and possible side effects. It may take time and perseverance to find the right drug or combination of drugs for you.

Not everybody needs medication, but your doctor will recommend it if you both think that it will help your symptoms of depression. Medications are more likely to be recommended if your depression is severe, long-lasting, or marked by deep sadness or if you have already had two episodes of depression. Medication is also used to treat people with depression who are experiencing hallucinations or delusions. If your depressive illness has responded well to medication in the past, your doctor will probably want to use it now. For some people, medication is their first choice of treatment. Others try it only if psychotherapy fails to ease their symptoms.

If this is your first episode of depression, you may take medication for about 9 months. If you have already had two episodes, you will probably take the medication for about 2 years. If this is your third or fourth episode, or if you have bipolar depression, your doctor may recommend medication indefinitely. Continuing medication can often prevent the depression from coming back.

You may not like the idea of medication. Taking pills to make yourself feel better may seem like a weakness. But many people use medication to control illness—for example, to control high blood pressure. Aspirin cannot cure arthritis, but it does ease pain. It is not a sign of weakness to take medication to control blood pressure or aspirin for arthritis, and neither is it a weakness to take medication for depression. Perhaps you fear medication will alter your personality. But depression has already affected your personality. If you are an artistic person, you may worry that medication will dampen your creativity. However, many doctors think that full mental health actually promotes creativity.

You may also be afraid of becoming dependent on medication. But medications that treat depressive illness are not addictive. You may also find it hard to accept that your body and mind are ill and that you need medication to get your health back. But medication may improve your ability to cope with life's hardships and can restore your good judgment.

In choosing a medication for you, your doctor will try to find one that will make you feel better without side effects or one that has side effects you can live with. Common side effects of antidepressants include dry mouth, feeling dizzy, constipation, drowsiness, and sleeping problems. More serious side effects include difficulty passing urine, palpitations, problems with sexual functioning, or seizures. Also, your doctor will ask whether a particular drug has helped you in the past and may choose that drug. The doctor may not select a medication that you have used before if you have developed another condition and are taking new medications that could interact badly with your old medication. In addition, other drugs that you need to take, such as medication for high blood pressure, your state of health, and your age, may affect the doctor's choice of medication. For example, older people and children may need different doses compared to young adults.

Beginning Your Medication

If your doctor recommends medication, ask any questions you want answered before you start taking the drug. The following are suggestions for questions to ask your doctor:

149

- What is the name of the medication?
- What dose will I need?
- What are the side effects of this medication?
- How will this medication help me?
- Are there other medications that could achieve the same effect?
- How much will this medication cost? Can I use a generic equivalent?
- When do I take this medication?
- Should I avoid certain foods while using this medication?
- Can I drink alcohol while using this medication?
- Should I avoid other medications while using this one?
- What should I do if I forget to take my medication? Should I take a double dose?
- How long will I need this medication?
- How likely is it that this medication will help me?
- How will I know if the medication is working?
- How soon should I feel better?

Once you begin taking the medication, it is very important to take the medication exactly as prescribed. If you miss a pill, do not take a double dose without checking with your doctor. If you experience side effects that interfere with your life or otherwise concern you, call your doctor right away. Do not wait for your scheduled visit to mention them. If you develop a rash while taking the medication, you are probably having an allergic reaction; call your doctor right away.

Depending on your type of illness and treatment, your doctor will schedule a follow-up visit after you start medication. The purpose of this follow-up visit is to determine how well the drug is working and to make any necessary adjustments. Your doctor will ask about your symptoms to make sure your depression is improving. If your depression is not subsiding, he or she will probably increase the dose of your medication.

Your doctor may ask detailed and personal questions about how any side effects are affecting your life. Say, for instance, that your medication has interfered with your ability to function sexually. If you are not currently sexually active, you may be willing to live with this problem for a time. If you are involved in a continuing sexual relationship, however, this may present a major problem. Your doctor can try to ease the side effects you are experiencing by adjusting your dose, by changing the time of day when you take the medication, by switching to a different drug, or by adding another medication.

During your visit, your doctor may draw a blood sample to check how much medication has built up in your blood. Some drugs start to take effect only after reaching a certain concentration level; the blood test shows how close you are to that point. The test is also used to confirm that you are taking the medication as prescribed.

If your doctor adjusts your medication—for example, by increasing the dose—another follow-up visit will take place a few weeks later. Once again, he or she will ask about your symptoms and side effects. If your depression is not improving, he or she may change your treatment in some way. For example, you may switch to a different medication or decide to get psychotherapy as well.

Your depressive illness may respond well to the first medication your doctor recommends, or you may have to try one after another. Sooner or later, most people find a medication or combination of medications that makes them feel well.

Doctors use several different kinds of medication to treat depressive illness. These drugs are classified according to which conditions they relieve. For example, drugs that relieve depression are called antidepressants. The selection of drugs that can treat depressive illness is constantly growing, increasing your chances of finding one that will alleviate your symptoms.

If you have major depression, you will probably be treated with an antidepressant. Antidepressants are divided into several categories, according to the effect they have on your brain chemistry. They include tricyclic antidepressants (TCAs), monoamine oxidase inhibitors (MAOIs), selective serotonin reuptake inhibitors (SSRIs), and other antidepressants.

If you have bipolar depression, you will probably be prescribed a mood-stabilizing drug, such as lithium. Mood stabilizers can treat both the depression and mania of bipolar illness. In addition, drugs used to treat seizures, or anticonvulsants, have been found to curb mania. People who have hallucinations or delusions may be treated with antipsychotic drugs, which are sometimes called neuroleptic medications. In addition, some people with mania use antianxiety drugs.

If you have dysthymia (chronic, mild depression), you may be treated with tricyclic antidepressants, MAOIs, SSRIs, bupropion, or a combination of these medications. Much remains to be learned about the treatment of dysthymia, but some doctors think MAOIs and SSRIs are the most effective medication for this disorder.

About 10 percent of people with dysthymia develop hypomania (mild mania) after taking antidepressants. Some doctors think dysthymia in these people may be related to bipolar depression in some way, since this reaction often occurs in people who have relatives with bipolar depression. If you develop hypomania, your doctor may try treating your illness with lithium, either alone or with antidepressants.

Your doctor may prescribe only one of these medications. Or you may take a combination of drugs to control your various symptoms.

Antidepressants

Antidepressants work by altering your brain's supply of neuro-transmitters, the chemical messengers used by the brain to send messages and regulate emotions. Chapter 3 discusses more fully how neurotransmitters work and the relationship between neuro-transmitters and depression. Briefly, neurotransmitters carry mes-sages across the gap, or synapse, between nerve cells, or neurons. The neurotransmitter completes its journey by docking in a re-ceptor on the receiving neuron. Once the neurotransmitters have completed their task, they float back into the synapse. There they will either be taken back by the sending neuron, a process called reuptake, or broken down by a substance called monoamine oxi-dase. Either way, the brain wipes the synapse clean of neurotrans-mitters.

Antidepressants improve your mood by interfering with this cleanup process. As explained in Chapter 3, doctors believe de-pression comes from having too much or too little of certain neurotransmitters—such as serotonin, norepinephrine, dopa-mine—and other chemical messengers that are involved in your emotional reactions. They think that one or more of these neuro-transmitters fail to dock on a neuron in the correct numbers. As a result, illness can develop. Antidepressants are believed to work by altering the balance of neurotransmitters zipping around your synapses, thus changing the chemistry to your advantage.

TRICYCLIC ANTIDEPRESSANTS

Tricyclic antidepressants (TCAs) are the drugs that have been used longest to treat depression. They get their name from their chemical structure, which consists of three rings. Like many medical breakthroughs, TCAs were discovered by accident. During the 1950s, a Swiss doctor tried giving a new medication, imipramine, to people with schizophrenia. Imipramine did little to control schizophrenia, but it did brighten the moods of the people who received it considerably. Before long, scientists realized that imipramine could lift depression.

Today, imipramine is still used to ease depression, under the brand names Janimine, Norfranil, Presamine, and Tofranil. It is only one of many tricyclic antidepressants. Others include amitriptyline (Endep, Elavil, Amitid), amoxapine (Asendin), clomipramine (Anafranil), desipramine (Norpramin, Pertofrane [Canada only at this writing]), doxepin (Adapin, Sinequan), maprotiline (Ludiomil), nortriptyline (Aventyl, Pamelor), and protriptyline (Vivactil).

If this is the first time you have used an antidepressant, your doctor may recommend a tricyclic antidepressant. Many doctors know tricyclics well and feel comfortable prescribing them because these drugs have been around longer than other antidepressants. Tricyclics also have a good track record of helping people with depression. Between 70 percent and 80 percent of seriously depressed people who take a TCA feel better. These drugs are also less expensive than newer antidepressants.

If you start taking a tricyclic antidepressant, you will not feel better right way. It usually takes several weeks to lift depression. Doctors do not fully understand why this is so. No two people respond in exactly the same way to a tricyclic. If you are like most, however, you will start sleeping better within a few days of starting the drug. Over the next few weeks, your other symptoms—such as anxiety, agitation, or hopelessness—will improve. Next, your interest in activities that used to be fun may return. Generally, your sadness will be the last symptom to leave.

Tricyclic antidepressants block the reuptake of norepinephrine, a mood-altering neurotransmitter, thereby increasing the amount of norepinephrine in your brain. Some also block reuptake of serotonin. Tricyclic antidepressants block reuptake almost immediately, but it may take several weeks for your mood to improve.

Unfortunately, tricyclic antidepressants also affect other neurotransmitters that help regulate certain body processes. This leads to side effects, which commonly include sleepiness or drowsiness. Side effects will vary depending on which TCA you take. Other possible side effects are dry mouth, constipation, difficulty urinating, vision problems, and a racing heart. Finally, you may feel lightheaded or dizzy when you stand up quickly, an effect called orthostatic hypotension. Less common side effects are rashes, sweating, tremors, delayed or reduced sexual orgasms, weight gain, and dry eyes. (If you wear soft contact lenses, you may notice that they feel gritty after you start taking a TCA.)

Always tell your doctor about any side effects you experience. Some side effects may subside as your body adjusts to the medication, or your doctor may be able to get rid of them by lowering the dose of your medication. You can also take steps to control those that linger. For example, you can make your mouth water with sugarless candy or gum and you can fight constipation by drinking more water and eating more fruit, vegetables, and whole grains. If your TCA makes you sleepy, your doctor may tell you to take it at night so that you get a good night's sleep.

If you do not feel better after several weeks on a TCA, your doctor may test your blood for levels of antidepressant medication. He or she may adjust your dose, which is often an effective step. Some people simply require a higher dose than others because their bodies differ in the way they process the drug.

TCAs are not for everyone. Because an overdose can be fatal, these drugs are seldom given to people who feel suicidal unless they are in the hospital. Also, people with certain disorders, such as coronary artery disease, cannot take TCAs because they may increase heart rate. In addition, people with bipolar depression cannot take tricyclics because antidepressant drugs can push them into hypomania or mania.

MONOAMINE OXIDASE INHIBITORS

Many doctors think monoamine oxidase inhibitors (MAOIs) are as good or better than TCAs at treating depression. These drugs are trickier to take, though, because you must avoid some foods, beverages, and medications while you are on them. Ignoring these restrictions can bring on severely elevated (high) blood pressure. If you can live with the inconvenience of the possible interactions, you may find MAOIs very helpful. They often work when other drugs have failed. MAOIs may be particularly effective in treating atypical depression, which involves oversleeping, overeating, and feeling worse in the evening than in the morning. Generally, your doctor will not suggest an MAOI as your first medication to try. If you have tried a TCA without success—this happens to about

1 person in 5—an MAOI may be right for you. Also, MAOIs can be used by certain people who cannot take TCAs, such as those with heart disease.

Monoamine oxidase inhibitors have been used since the 1950s. As with tricyclic antidepressants, their ability to ease depression was discovered by accident. Doctors noticed that a drug called iproniazid, which was then used to combat tuberculosis, was making people feel happy and cheerful. The drug, which was an MAOI, became popular as a treatment for depression. Later, however, the drug had to be withdrawn from the market when it was shown to cause health problems in many people. Today, two MAOI drugs are sold in the US: phenelzine sulfate (Nardil) and tranylcypromine sulfate (Parnate).

Like most antidepressants, MAOIs begin to relieve your symptoms only after you have been taking them for several weeks. Their common side effects include dizziness, changes in blood pressure, weight gain, sleepiness or insomnia, difficulty in reaching sexual orgasm, and puffy ankles and fingers. Sometimes, but not often, they cause dry mouth, constipation, blurred vision, and difficulty in urinating. MAOIs can also bring on hypomania in some people, including people with bipolar depression. The side effects you have a chance of experiencing vary depending on which MAOI you take. Phenelzine sulfate is more likely to cause weight gain, for example, but tranylcypromine sulfate seems to cause more insomnia. While an overdose of MAOIs can be fatal if they are combined with certain other substances, these drugs are less lethal than TCAs by themselves.

Monoamine oxidase inhibitors help you feel better by preventing monamine oxidase, a substance found in nerve endings, from doing its job. As explained in Chapter 3, monamine oxidase breaks down the neurotransmitters norepinephrine, dopamine, and serotonin, all of which have an effect on your mood. When you take an MAOI, fewer of these neurotransmitters are broken down, leaving you with a larger supply and an improved mood.

This disruption of monoamine oxidase is why you must avoid certain foods, drinks, and medications while using MAOIs. One of monoamine oxidase's other jobs is to break down a substance called tyramine, which can raise your blood pressure. Normally, if you ate a food containing tyramine, monoamine oxidase would get rid of it long before it could affect blood pressure. If you take an MAOI, however, that does not happen. Tyramine can then flood your system, raise your blood pressure significantly, and cause throbbing headaches, nausea, vomiting, stroke, heart attack, or death.

Thus, you must avoid consuming anything containing tyramine while you are on this medication. The list of foods with tyramine is quite long. It includes:

- Aged cheese and foods made with it, such as pizza
- Sour cream
- Fermented sausage, such as pepperoni or salami
- Pastrami and corned beef
- Tofu
- Soy sauce and teriyaki
- Salted, pickled, or smoked fish
- Caviar (fish eggs)
- Escargot (snails)
- Sauerkraut and pickles
- Fava beans, lima beans, Italian beans, and Chinese pea pods
- Yeast products, such as brewer's yeast

- Avocados
- Dried figs

In addition, you must avoid certain beverages, including Chianti wine, champagne, beer, nonalcoholic beer, whiskey, and some liqueurs. You must also avoid large quantities of other alcoholic drinks, sour cream, chocolate, and caffeinated coffee, tea, or soft drinks.

Never take another medication with an MAOI without discussing it with your doctor first; the combination may cause a severe, life-threatening reaction. Among the medications you should avoid are nonprescription cold remedies; nasal decongestants, nose drops, and cough remedies; most sinus, allergy, hay fever, and asthma medications; some local anesthetics; and some prescription pain medications, such as Demerol.

If you take an MAOI, you should learn to recognize the signs of high blood pressure. If you experience them—a headache at the back of the neck, a stiff neck, a pounding heart, nausea, vomiting, or collapse—go to your doctor's office or a hospital emergency department. In addition, consider wearing a medical alert bracelet or carry a medical alert card in your wallet.

SELECTIVE SEROTONIN REUPTAKE INHIBITORS

Selective serotonin reuptake inhibitors (SSRIs) are newer drugs that have become popular weapons against depression. Some doctors think SSRIs have fewer or less problematic side effects than do TCAs or MAOIs. If this is your first time taking an antidepressant, your doctor may recommend an SSRI. One drawback to these drugs is that they tend to be more expensive than other antidepressants. SSRIs include fluoxetine (Prozac), paroxetine (Paxil), fluvoxamine (Luvox), and sertraline (Zoloft).

Fluoxetine was the first SSRI found to be effective in treating depression and has achieved great popularity. Since it was introduced in the 1980s, fluoxetine has become the world's most widely prescribed antidepressant. This drug is popular for many reasons. For many people, it causes fewer side effects than do TCAs or MAOIs. While TCAs can make you gain weight, for example, fluoxetine may cause a small weight loss. Fluoxetine is simple to use, with dosage sometimes consisting of only one pill a day. In addition, you cannot overdose on fluoxetine.

SSRIs work by increasing your brain's supply of the mood-regulating neurotransmitter serotonin. They do this by blocking the reuptake (reabsorption) of serotonin in the synapse. Because SSRIs target only serotonin and do not affect other brain chemicals, they tend to cause fewer side effects than do older antidepressants. As with other antidepressants, it may take 3 to 5 weeks to feel better when you are taking SSRIs. Many people, however, say they feel better much more quickly, often within a few days.

Common side effects for SSRIs include insomnia, nervousness, agitation, nausea, diarrhea, and headaches. Less common are sleepiness, yawning, heavy sweating, and rashes. One disturbing side effect is possible sexual difficulties, including lack of interest, arousal problems, and difficulty achieving orgasm. Your side effects may subside after your body adjusts to the drug. If they do not, your doctor may add another drug to counter the side effect, lower your dose, or switch you to a different SSRI.

SSRIs are not for everyone. People with bipolar depression should not take these drugs because they can bring on hypomania or mania. Because SSRIs are chemically processed in the liver, people with liver disease, such as hepatitis, cannot use them. Fluoxetine has been suspected of making some people suicidal or aggressive and has received some bad publicity as a result. Although one small study found a link between fluoxetine and suicidal thoughts and behavior, larger, better-controlled studies have not found a connection.

OTHER ANTIDEPRESSANTS

Several other antidepressants available today are different in chemical makeup or action than the categories already described. These drugs include bupropion (Wellbutrin), trazodone (Desyrel), and such newer drugs as venlafaxine hydrochloride (Effexor), nefazodone hydrochloride (Serzone), and mirtazapine (Remeron).

Bupropion is less likely than other antidepressants to cause weight gain and sexual problems. It also seems less likely to bring on mania or hypomania in people with bipolar depression. Among the side effects you may notice while taking this drug are excitement, agitation, sleeplessness, nausea, and a slight shaking, or tremor. Bupropion is believed to work by blocking reuptake of the neurotransmitter dopamine.

Bupropion can cause seizures in high doses; in fact, it was withdrawn from the market for a period of time. To minimize your risk, your doctor will probably advise you to take this medication in small amounts two or three times a day.

Trazodone is believed to work by blocking reuptake of the neurotransmitter serotonin. Trazodone may also have a few side effects; among those you may notice are digestive problems, a bad taste in your mouth, nausea, or a rapid heartbeat. Trazodone may also make your blood pressure drop slightly. Because this drug can cause abnormal heart rhythms, it is not given to people with heart disease. On very rare occasions, trazodone can give a man painful and long-lasting erections, which is a serious and possibly dangerous side effect.

Venlafaxine hydrochloride is a kind of antidepressant called a selective serotonin noradrenergic reuptake inhibitor (SSNRI). It blocks reuptake of the mood-regulating neurotransmitters serotonin, norepinephrine, and dopamine but does not interfere with other brain chemicals. Its possible side effects include headaches, sleepiness, and dizziness.

Nefazodone hydrochloride increases the amount of serotonin and norepinephrine available. Its possible side effects include sleepiness, low blood pressure, and blurred vision.

A different kind of antidepressant, mirtazapine, was approved for sale in 1996. Mirtazapine works by stimulating the release of serotonin and norepinephrine while also blocking two receptors for serotonin. Mirtazapine seems less likely to bring on sexual problems but may cause drowsiness, increased appetite, weight gain, and dizziness.

Mood-Stabilizing Medications

Mood-stabilizing medications are used to stabilize the shifting high and low moods of people with bipolar depression. Lithium is the primary drug in this category. Anticonvulsant drugs, usually used to control seizures, have also been shown to be useful in helping some people stabilize their moods. These drugs include carbamazepine (Tegretol), valproic acid (Depakene), divalproex sodium (Depakote), and clonazepam (Klonopin).

LITHIUM

Lithium is used to treat both the depression and the mania of bipolar illness. In addition, many people with bipolar depression take lithium when they are feeling well because it seems to prevent new episodes. Lithium can ease sadness during depression, curb euphoria during mania, and maintain equilibrium during normal times. If you have bipolar depression, you may take lithium alone or with other drugs.

Lithium comes from a mineral found in tiny amounts in the human body, plants, mineral springs, and rocks. As a medication, it is usually found in the form of a salt, as lithium carbonate or lithium citrate. Lithium is sold under several brand names, including Eskalith, Lithobid, and Cibalith-S. It is available in tablets, capsules, and a liquid.

Like many drugs used to treat depressive illness, lithium was discovered by accident. Lithium's debut in the early 1940s, as a salt substitute for people on low-sodium diets, was a disaster. The doses used were too high, and some people were poisoned and even died. In 1949, an Australian researcher noticed that guinea pigs treated with lithium remained calm, even if they were prodded or poked. By the 1960s, lithium was used in several countries to treat bipolar illness, but the US held back until 1974. Today, many people live normal lives thanks to this drug.

Lithium does not work for everybody. About 1 in 5 people with bipolar depression are not helped by it. Your kidneys eliminate this drug and prevent it from building up to toxic levels within your body; thus, people with damaged kidneys can take it only with special precautions. Also, lithium does little for certain types of bipolar depression (see Chapter 2), such as rapid cycling, in which people have frequent episodes of illness (4 or more per year).

Even if lithium works for you, be careful to take the medication as prescribed. Too little lithium may be useless, and too much may be lethal. Doctors will order regular blood tests to check the level of lithium in your blood. At first, your blood will be checked every few days. Then after you have been taking lithium for a while, your blood will be checked less frequently, perhaps every few months. Your kidneys will also be tested from time to time to make sure they can excrete lithium from your body. Your doctor will also check your thyroid gland, because lithium can enlarge the gland or make it sluggish.

Once you start taking lithium, you should feel better in about 10 days to 2 weeks. Because your body metabolizes lithium very quickly, you may need to take the drug two to four times a day. If you were to take your entire daily dose at once, the level of lithium in your blood might be too high. Lithium is available in some forms that release the drug into your body more slowly. If you opt for one of these, you can take the drug less frequently. However, these forms of lithium, sold under such brand names as Lithobid and Eskalith CR, are more expensive than others.

About 40 percent of people taking lithium experience side effects at first. These include digestive problems, such as nausea, vomiting, diarrhea, and stomachaches. Your hands may tremble slightly and you may feel exhausted, weak, or confused. You may be extremely thirsty or need to urinate often. Some of these side effects usually ease after a few days, but the trembling hands, thirst, and excessive urination may persist. Your doctor may be able to help by lowering your dose of the drug, but make certain that you talk to the doctor before deciding to lower the dose.

In addition, some people gain weight while on lithium. Watching your calories and increasing your exercise can guard against this. A small percentage of people develop hypothyroidism. This seems to affect women more than men. Acne and dry skin are common problems. Rare side effects include a bad taste in your mouth, memory loss, and hair loss.

Because a buildup of lithium in your body could harm or kill you, you should never take more than your usual dose, even to make up for forgetting an earlier one. Certain medications, including the antibiotic tetracycline and such nonsteroidal anti-inflammatory painkillers as aspirin and ibuprofen, can also increase the levels of lithium in your blood. Talk to your doctor before taking any other medication. It is a good idea to ask your doctor about alcohol also, because this can react with lithium and make you confused.

You cannot start on a low-sodium diet after you have started taking lithium; your kidneys need sodium to excrete it from your body. If your body has too little sodium, lithium will build up and could poison you. Call your doctor whenever you become dehydrated from vomiting or having diarrhea. He or she will probably advise you to take a lower dose of lithium at such times.

No one understands exactly how lithium works. One theory is that it affects the brain's system of sending messages. When you feel happy, sad, angry, or have any other emotional reaction, your brain sends messages throughout its network of neurons. Lithium seems to have some effect on the complex reactions that take place inside each neuron as a message passes through it. These reactions may be overactive during mania and depression, and lithium may slow them down. Another theory is that lithium blocks a protein that helps regulate certain neurotransmitters. But no one knows for sure.

Although lithium is used primarily to treat bipolar depression, your doctor may prescribe it for major depression if he or she cannot find an antidepressant that works. In some cases, lithium taken with an antidepressant makes the antidepressant more effective. This treatment is called lithium augmentation.

Talk to your doctor about how long you should take lithium. If your illness is very mild, you may take it for only 6 months or so. But many people take lithium indefinitely in order to prevent relapses, especially if they have had two or more severe episodes within a 5-year period.

ANTICONVULSANT MEDICATIONS

Several drugs originally developed to treat seizures also help control bipolar depression. These drugs, called anticonvulsants, subdue mania and may prevent future episodes. Anticonvulsants include carbamazepine, valproic acid, divalproex sodium, and clonazepam. Your doctor may prescribe one of these drugs, either alone or with lithium. In addition, you may take an anticonvulsant if you have a severe form of bipolar depression, such as mixed state depression or rapid cycling (see Chapter 2).

Carbamazepine. Carbamazepine has helped many people with severe bipolar depression. About 80 percent of those who try this drug feel better. Doctors think that when an amino acid called gamma-aminobutyric acid (GABA) is attached to these neurons, it blocks other chemicals that ordinarily stimulate the limbic system. In the same way, it also calms nerves that control muscle movement and thus helps prevent seizures. By interfering in this way, carbamazepine makes your moods less extreme.

Before you start taking carbamazepine, your doctor will perform a blood test to make sure your liver can handle the drug safely. In high doses, carbamazepine can damage certain parts of your body, including the liver and blood. In rare cases, carbamazepine can stop your bone marrow from producing blood cells. If this happens, your life could be in danger.

When you start on the medication, your doctor will probably begin with a low dose and gradually increase it. Your doctor will regularly test your blood, frequently in the beginning and at regular intervals later, to ensure that your bone marrow is functioning properly and that the carbamazepine does not reach dangerously high levels in your system.

People usually take carbamazepine twice a day. Because of the risk of poisoning, ask your doctor what to do if you miss a dose. This is one medication you should not keep in the bathroom cabinet, because humidity can make it less powerful. Instead, keep it in a dark, cool, dry place.

While taking carbamazepine, you may feel dizzy, drowsy, or confused. You may find that you walk less steadily than usual. Make sure you understand how this drug affects you before you drive a car or operate machinery. Also, some people complain of headaches, double vision, nausea, diarrhea, and rash. Many of these side effects may subside after a week or so. Carbamazepine also affects the action of other medications, so be sure to tell your doctor about all prescription and nonprescription medications that you are on. It makes birth control pills less effective, so you should plan on using a second or alternate method. It may decrease the effect of some drugs and increase the effect of others. Ask your doctor about other medications before using carbamazepine.

Valproic acid and divalproex sodium. Two similar anticonvulsants, valproic acid (Depakene) and divalproex sodium (Depakote), also help about 80 percent of the people who try them. They help subdue mania and either prevent future mood swings or make them less severe. Doctors may prescribe one of these drugs for you if you did not find lithium or carbamazepine helpful or if their side effects were too uncomfortable. As with many other depression medications, you may have to take them for several weeks before noticing a difference.

These drugs have their own set of side effects. They may make you drowsy at first and they may cause such digestive problems as stomach upset or diarrhea. Some people also find that some of their hair falls out. These side effects usually go away after a few weeks.

High amounts of valproic acid or divalproex sodium can damage your liver. Your doctor will test your liver before you start the drug to make sure it is safe for you. In addition, your blood will be tested periodically to make sure blood levels of the drug are safe. You may receive a blood test every week at first. These medications can react with other drugs, including other anticonvulsants and alcohol, causing changes in blood level. Talk to your doctor before taking any other medication or before having an alcoholic drink with these drugs.

Clonazepam. The anticonvulsant clonazepam also relieves some symptoms of mania. This drug does not even out your mood like lithium or other anticonvulsants, but it eases some of mania's effects. For example, it can relieve your racing thoughts, pressured speech, and hyperactivity. You may receive this drug in the early part of your treatment for bipolar depression because it often works more quickly than lithium. Side effects of clonazepam include dizziness, sleepiness, clumsiness, and psychological and/or physical dependence.

Antipsychotic Drugs

Antipsychotic drugs, also called neuroleptics, treat people who have lost touch with reality, a disorder called psychosis. Your doctor may prescribe an antipsychotic medication if you have a delusion or hallucination during mania or depression. These drugs also help relieve psychosis in people with psychotic depression (see Chapter 2).

Among the commonly used antipsychotic drugs are chlorpromazine (Thorazine), haloperidol (Haldol), and the newer drugs clozapine (Clozaril), olanzapine (Zyprexa), and risperidone (Risperdol). If you develop psychosis with depression, you will take an antipsychotic drug in addition to an antidepressant. When your psychosis lifts, the antipsychotic medication can be tapered and stopped. Antipsychotic drugs can be taken as tablet, liquid, or injection. They help about 60 percent of the people who take them.

While you are taking an antipsychotic medication, you may experience constipation, blurred vision, sleepiness, or dry mouth. These side effects may disappear as you get used to the drug. You are also likely to have problems with your muscles and with movement. For example, you may have muscle contractions that cause involuntary movements of your face, neck, tongue, back, and eyes. Doctors call this a dystonic reaction. Or your movements may become stiff, a condition called akinesia. Or, you may be unable to sit still, a condition called akathisia. If you have these muscle problems, your doctor may treat them with a second drug or change your antipsychotic medication.

A more extreme side effect is tardive dyskinesia, which causes permanent, involuntary movements of the mouth, head, and body. This generally happens after a person has taken the drug for more than a year. The lower your dose of antipsychotic, the less risk you have of developing tardive dyskinesia. Other side effects include menstrual changes in women, sexual problems, weight gain, and sensitivity to the sun.

Antipsychotic drugs are believed to work by altering your brain chemistry to lessen the effect of the neurotransmitter dopamine. Because antipsychotic drugs work in this way, doctors think excess dopamine or overactive dopamine receptors may produce psychotic symptoms.

Antianxiety Drugs

Antianxiety drugs, also called sedatives or hypnotics, are sometimes used to treat mania or depression. During mania, you may receive a sedative called lorazepam (Ativan). This can ease some parts of mania, such as racing thoughts, pressured speech, and hyperactivity. This drug acts quickly, and your doctor may prescribe it while you are waiting for another medication to take effect. In addition, you can develop psychological and/or physical dependence on this and other antianxiety drugs if taken for more than a few weeks.

The antianxiety drug alprazolam (Xanax) is sometimes used to treat depression. This drug can also act quickly but is usually used for only a short time because it is addictive. You may receive this drug if your depression is not severe yet needs immediate attention and if health problems (such as heart disease) rule out antidepressants. If you have a history of substance abuse, you will not be given this drug.

Choosing the Right Medication

Finding the right medication for depressive illness is difficult for some people. Older people may have medical conditions that rule out certain drugs. In addition, they may take other medications that can interfere with antidepressants. Certain side effects are also more serious in older people. For example, dizziness is generally more dangerous in an older person because a fall can cause serious injuries. Some antidepressants can also affect the heart, making them dangerous for older people with heart damage. In addition, the bodies of older people may break down these drugs more slowly than do the bodies of younger adults. Sometimes the medication can build up in the bloodstream of older people, causing confusion and memory problems.

Women who want to become pregnant may also have difficulty finding proper medication. In general, doctors recommend that pregnant women avoid medications to make sure the fetus develops normally. Some medications used to treat depressive illness may damage the fetus. For example, babies whose mothers used valproic acid or divalproex sodium during pregnancy may have stunted growth, unusually small heads, and facial abnormalities. In addition, this drug increases the baby's risk of spina bifida, a birth defect in which the spinal column does not form properly. Lithium may cause heart defects in a fetus, although the drug's role in such defects is still controversial and not yet proven. Some medications may be safer during pregnancy than others. If you take medication, talk to your doctor before trying to become pregnant.

Nursing mothers may also find it difficult to select an antidepressant, since many of these drugs pass into breast milk. If you are breast-feeding, ask your doctor about the dangers your medication poses to your baby.

If you have a medical condition, your choice of antidepressants may be limited. If you have heart disease, for example, your doctor will probably steer you away from TCAs because they can affect your heart. You are more likely to be treated with trazodone, bupropion, nefazodone hydrochloride, or an SSRI.

Only since the 1980s have doctors recognized that children and adolescents can develop depressive illness. As a result, medications for depressive illness were not developed with young people in mind, and their effects on growing bodies are unknown. In general, few medications have been tested on children, including antidepressants and lithium. Among those tested, some researchers have found that fluoxetine (Prozac) may help young people, while TCAs may be less helpful. Nevertheless, many children and adolescents receive these medications, often with good results.

Problems With Medication

Sometimes treating depressive illness with medication does not go smoothly. Most people see improvement within 3 weeks, but if you do not, your doctor may change your medication in some way by the fourth week. For example, he or she may increase your dose, supplement the drug with another, or try a different medication. In very rare instances, people may remain depressed despite medication. If this happens to you, your doctor will then probably continue to tackle your illness with new combinations of drugs until the right mixture of drugs is found.

Sometimes your doctor will revise your diagnosis if the treatment has no effect. Or he or she may suggest a different kind of treatment in addition to medication, such as ECT or psychotherapy (see pages 175 through 185).

If medication is not effective, your doctor may have prescribed too low a dose or may not have tried all the different medications available. Some doctors still regard depressive illness as a primarily psychological disorder and may have mixed feelings about treating it with medication, even though there is research proving that altering brain chemistry can help people with depression. Discuss with your doctor his or her position on other medications; if you are still interested in trying other prescriptions that your doctor will not give you, consider getting a referral to another doctor.

Sometimes medication is ineffective because you do not take it as prescribed. Doctors call this noncompliance. Of the people admitted to the hospital for depression, 20 percent to 25 percent had failed to take their medication. You may have all sorts of reasons for not following your doctor's instructions, but this is not a good idea. You may think a larger dose will be more powerful or a smaller dose will have fewer side effects. Maybe you take your medication only when you feel bad and stop as soon as you improve, despite the fact that you need to take it daily. The symptoms of your illness, such as forgetfulness or hopelessness, may also affect whether you pay attention to your doctor's instructions. In addition, you may resent having to depend on a pill to feel well. No matter how good your reason for changing your dose, a medication is effective only when taken as prescribed.

LIGHT THERAPY

Light therapy, also called phototherapy, is used to treat people with SAD, a type of depression that occurs in the winter. People who receive light therapy sit in front of extremely bright lights for a certain length of time every day. Doctors think light therapy works by compensating for the loss of sunlight during winter, which is thought to trigger SAD. Light therapy helps about three fourths of the people with SAD.

You may need between 30 minutes and several hours of light therapy a day to shake your depression. Several companies make special lights you can use at home, under the direction of your doctor. These may be ordinary white fluorescent lights, but about 20 times brighter than those in your kitchen. Some researchers believe full-spectrum lights, which most closely imitate the light of the sun, are more helpful. The lights used must be specially filtered to block out ultraviolet rays, which can cause cataracts. Do not try to give yourself light therapy without guidance from a doctor.

Generally, light therapy improves your mood within 3 to 14 days. Some researchers think this therapy works best in the early morning, but many people find this inconvenient because it cuts in on time needed for family and work. Your doctor may advise you to use the lights at the best time for you. If your depression does not improve, you might want to try a different time. Some people try to make use of their time in front of the lights by reading or writing. Side effects are uncommon with light therapy, but some people experience headaches, eyestrain, irritability, and insomnia.

Some researchers are experimenting with new kinds of light therapy. One example is an artificial dawn simulated by an electric device that you attach to your bedside lamp. Several hours before you normally wake in the morning, the lamp will switch itself on, but at very low levels of light. The dim light gradually increases, simulating dawn. This artificial dawn has helped some people with SAD. Researchers do not fully understand how artificial dawn works, but they have noted a link between SAD and disturbed circadian (sleep–wake) rhythms (see Chapter 3).

If light therapy fails to alleviate your illness, your doctor may recommend that you change your lifestyle to head off future bouts of depression. For example, you might make a special effort to walk outside on sunny days or you might try taking winter vacations in sunny locations.

ELECTROCONVULSIVE THERAPY

If you are severely depressed and cannot take medication, you may be treated with ECT, also known as shock treatment, an effective and fast-acting treatment for depression and mania. About 80 percent of people with depression or mania feel better after receiving ECT. The treatment is at least as powerful as medication, perhaps more so, and it works faster. But because it uses electricity directly on the brain, it is used mainly for people who do have problems with medication; who are severely depressed, manic, psychotic, or suicidal; or whose disease has not responded to other treatments.

Before ECT, you will receive an anesthetic that will sedate you for a short period of time so that you do not remember or feel the treatment. During the treatment, electrodes placed on your head pass low electrical currents through one or both sides of your brain. When the currents pass through one side, the treatment is called unilateral ECT. When the currents pass through both sides, the treatment is called bilateral ECT. These currents bring about an episode of uncontrolled electrical activity in the brain called a seizure. Seizures can cause tingling and twitching movements, among other symptoms. Because seizures can cause muscle contractions and stiff, jerking movements, you will also be given a short-acting muscle relaxant so that your body remains relaxed during your seizure. Your seizure will last anywhere from 25 seconds to about a minute. After the seizure passes, you will remain unconscious for about 10 to 15 minutes.

ECT is usually given three times a week. After 2 or 3 weeks, your depression or mania will lift. One theory about ECT presumes that the electrical shocks affect the parts of the brain that regulate your moods. It may also stimulate the brain's production of certain amino acids, which are the first step in producing neurotransmitters, the chemical messengers that can affect moods.

Unfortunately, the effect of ECT may be only temporary. About half of the people who receive it relapse within 6 months. To prevent relapse, your doctor may prescribe antidepressants or lithium after ECT. Side effects of ECT include confusion and memory loss, which usually last only a short time.

Many people are reluctant to receive ECT because of its checkered history. In the mid-20th century, ECT techniques were still unrefined, and people received high-energy currents while they were awake. Their bodies went into convulsions, sometimes breaking bones or stopping the heart. Often, ECT was performed against their will. Today, doctors take precautions at every step of the procedure to ensure a person's safety and well-being. Still, ECT remains controversial to many people.

PSYCHOTHERAPY

Psychotherapy, often referred to just as therapy, is a common treatment for depressive illness, either by itself or with medication. Psychotherapy consists of meeting with a therapist, either alone or as part of a group, to discuss your feelings, problems, and life experiences. Many kinds of health-care providers offer psychotherapy, including psychiatrists, psychologists, and social workers.

Therapists use many different techniques and approaches; these all stem from different theories about the causes of mental illness. Therapists who believe that depression stems mainly from negative thinking focus on changing such thoughts. Others say depression comes from faulty behavior developed in response to stress. Still others think depression is the result of unresolved childhood losses (see Chapter 3). One or several of these theories may influence your therapist's technique.

Psychotherapy has helped many people with depressive illness, either alone or with medication. Alone, some forms of psychotherapy are effective in easing mild to moderate depression in about 50 percent of people who have it. Even if your illness requires medication, you may find psychotherapy helpful. For example, psychotherapy can help you resolve mixed feelings about relying on medication to feel well. If you have bipolar depression, you are more likely to take your medication if you also participate in therapy. In addition, researchers have found that manic people who participate in psychotherapy are less likely to have a relapse.

Psychotherapy can help you assess the effect depressive illness has had on your life. Your illness may have strained your relationships and caused others to see you as unreliable. Knowing you are ill has probably changed your idea of yourself. You may wonder what you should tell your boss, children, and friends about your illness. Psychotherapy can help you resolve such issues.

Some doctors criticize psychotherapy because it is difficult to test with the same degree of scientific precision with which medications have been tested. However, two kinds of therapy—interpersonal therapy and cognitive therapy—have been shown by researchers to help depression. Psychotherapy also has other downfalls. Some forms can last for years, making it expensive, especially because many health insurance policies do not cover psychotherapy or limit their coverage of it. On the positive side, psychotherapy has none of the physical side effects of medication.

Your doctor may recommend psychotherapy instead of medication if your illness is mild to moderate, has lasted only a short time, and is not recurrent. In addition, if you are keen on psychotherapy or found it helpful in the past, your doctor will probably suggest you take part in it. You may decide to try psychotherapy if you cannot or will not take medication or if medication has not helped. Psychotherapy may also help you to cope if your daily life is very stressful.

Your doctor may recommend psychotherapy with medication if your illness is severe or has come back several times without entirely lifting in between. Also, if medication alone or psychotherapy alone has not worked, your doctor will probably suggest trying both. People with personality disorders may also be advised to try both treatments.

Psychotherapy will probably take longer than medication to have an effect. You should start to feel better after about 6 weeks. If you experience improvement but still have some symptoms after 12 weeks, ask your doctor when to expect further improvement.

There are many kinds of psychotherapy. Those thought to be particularly helpful in treating depressive illness include cognitive therapy, interpersonal therapy, and behavior therapy. Depending on your personal situation, psychodynamic therapy, family therapy, couples therapy, or any combination of therapies may also be used.

Cognitive Therapy

Cognitive therapy is a technique developed by American psychologist Aaron Beck that focuses on improving your self-image and your view of the world. If you are depressed, you may see yourself as a failure or a bad person. You may regard your situation as unbearably difficult or believe that nothing will ever improve. Cognitive therapists believe that if you learn to stop such thinking patterns, you will feel better. Your therapist will help you spot negative thoughts and test their validity, guide you in developing new ways of thinking, and rehearse new responses to situations.

Cognitive therapists believe that our thoughts are influenced by beliefs that we develop from childhood on. Depressed people are influenced by negative beliefs that they have developed about themselves or their actions. They develop such negative beliefs because they typically make one or more of the following mistakes in the way they think:

- They draw unreasonable conclusions, such as deciding they are to blame for everything that goes wrong.
- They base conclusions on one detail taken out of context.
- They base conclusions on one or two isolated pieces of information.
- They build up bad events and minimize the good ones.
- They take events personally, even when doing so is unreasonable.
- They see everything as black or white.

For cognitive therapists, moods are created by thought. If you feel depressed, you are thinking in a way that causes emotional pain. As you learn to think more objectively, the theory goes, you will feel better. Most cognitive therapists see this learning as a project that both of you work on together. Usually, the two of you will draw up a list of problems and goals and continue to work on the list.

Your therapist will try to teach you to question the automatic, negative thoughts that feed your depression. He or she may do this in a variety of ways. You might be asked to jot down these thoughts and bring the list to therapy. Or your therapist may challenge your dim view of yourself and your life by devising a daily schedule of activities. After you complete each activity, you will rate how much you enjoyed it and how well you handled it. These ratings may contradict your feeling that nothing fun ever happens and that you do nothing well. Or your therapist may use role reversal, defending your negative thoughts while you challenge them.

Cognitive therapy is often short, running about 12 to 16 sessions. However, if you have a long-lasting form of depression, such as dysthymia, your treatment may take anywhere from 6 months to 2 years.

Research has shown that cognitive therapy helps about 50 percent of the people who participate. Some researchers, however, believe that a combination of cognitive therapy and medication is better than either treatment on its own. Separate studies show that people with bipolar depression who receive cognitive therapy have fewer episodes of illness than do those who receive no psychotherapy. Doctors believe cognitive therapy has this effect because it helps people accept their ongoing need for medication.

Interpersonal Therapy

Interpersonal therapy is a technique that works to change the personal relationships that may contribute to your depression.

According to this theory, which was developed by psychiatrist Gerald Klerman and psychologist Myrna Weissman, such problems stem from difficulties in your personal relationships.

Your interpersonal therapist will try to improve your image of yourself and your communication skills, which in turn can make your relationships healthier. In your discussions, you will examine your ability to form and keep healthy relationships, your skill at handling new roles in life, and any prolonged grief you may be feeling. In this way, you and your therapist will identify the problems in your relationships and try to set them right.

Research has shown that interpersonal therapy helps about 50 percent of those who try it. This therapy may be less helpful in treating severe depression, although some research suggests that it may be the best choice for severely depressed people who refuse medication.

Interpersonal therapy generally lasts 12 to 16 weeks. This technique may not be widely available in all areas.

Behavior Therapy

Behavior therapy, also called behavioral or behavior modification therapy, helps you change actions that may aggravate your depression. The theory behind this therapy is that your depression is a kind of behavior, which you can both learn and unlearn. This idea comes mainly from the work done by Russian psychologist Ivan Pavlov during the 1920s and 1930s. Research shows that behavior therapy can relieve depression in about 50 percent of people who participate in it.

Behavior therapists believe you get depressed if too much is demanded of you and the rewards you receive are inadequate.

Your behavior therapist may refer to your rewards as positive reinforcement. For example, if you are an ambitious student but fall behind because of a learning disability, you might become depressed. Your behavior therapist will try to teach you how to make sure you receive sufficient rewards.

In some kinds of therapy, the therapist is there to mainly listen. By contrast, behavior therapists take a more active role. Your therapist will probably design an individual treatment plan for you, which takes into account the kind of depression you have and what may have caused it.

The behavioral therapist will probably not explore the psychological origins of your depression but will teach you to avoid behavior that causes depression. For example, if you often procrastinate, you may end up feeling depressed because procrastination does not take the task away. Instead, it makes the job at hand more difficult and postpones your reward for finishing. You and your therapist may tackle your procrastination in several ways. You may record every time you procrastinate in a journal or on a graph. Or, you may imagine yourself in the future at a time when you no longer procrastinate. You may learn to redirect thoughts that encourage procrastination. You may even wear a rubber band on your wrist that you will snap whenever you procrastinate.

Psychodynamic Therapy/Psychoanalysis

Psychodynamic therapy is based on the theory that a person's past experiences and unconscious wishes and fears have a strong effect upon his or her emotions and behavior. Many mental illnesses, the theory states, can be treated by giving an individual new insight into the workings of his or her mind and emotions.

This method of therapy requires more time than others, but it is also more ambitious. Rather than simply alleviating your symptoms, psychodynamic therapy tries to change your personality or character by helping you trust others, build intimacy with others, cope better with life, grieve unacknowledged losses, and experience a wide range of emotions.

According to psychodynamic theory, conflict between unconscious and conscious thoughts, beliefs, and wishes may cause depression. You may deal with uncomfortable conflicts by repressing them or unknowingly moving them from your conscious mind into your unconscious mind. The goal of psychodynamic therapy is to bring repressed and unresolved conflicts, often reaching back as far as childhood, into your conscious mind so that you can confront and heal them.

Your therapist may use several techniques to bring your repressed conflicts to light. You may be asked to relax and talk about anything that comes to mind, which can provide a glimpse into the workings of your unconscious mind. Your psychoanalyst may try to help you explore your dreams, which are seen as the product of your unconscious mind. You may be asked to describe your life, especially childhood memories. In addition, you may be asked to analyze your emotional reactions to the therapist, which may mimic your reactions to other people.

Psychodynamic therapy is based on the theories and techniques of Austrian physician Sigmund Freud. He invented the oldest form of psychodynamic therapy, called psychoanalysis. This intensive, long-term therapy (three or more sessions a week for 3 to 5 years) attempts to thoroughly examine all the aspects of your personality. By gaining deep insight, the theory states, you are able to make significant changes in your personality and behavior. The therapist, called a psychoanalyst, remains neutral; he or she does not try to offer solutions to day-to-day problems. Thus, psychoanalysis may not be appropriate if you are in a crisis or severely depressed or if you are experiencing symptoms of mania or psychosis.

In other forms of psychodynamic therapy, the therapist will offer you more active and direct support. In brief dynamic psychotherapy, treatment is focused on a specific problem and limited in duration, usually to a few months.

Psychodynamic therapy has several drawbacks. It may be expensive and take several years. The process of examining painful and hidden emotions may make you anxious and distressed at times. To take full advantage of this therapy, you need to be able to talk to and form relationships with other people and be motivated enough to apply the therapeutic insights to the rest of your life. There have been no objective research studies designed to test whether psychodynamic therapy is an effective treatment for depression. Yet even its critics acknowledge that psychodynamic therapy has helped many people with a variety of personality and other problems.

Family Therapy

Family therapy tries to teach your family members about your illness and shows them how they can help in your treatment. Families can be a great source of strength to a depressed person, provided they understand the illness and take part in its treatment.

During family therapy, you and your family members will meet with a therapist about five to ten times over a short period. You will discuss how your illness has changed your family's ideas about you and the roles family members play. Your family will learn the symptoms of your illness, discuss the possibility of its returning, learn the signs of a new episode, and examine treatment options. In addition, your family will discuss the chances of other members' becoming ill, since inheritance seems to play a role in depression.

Research has shown that some people with major depression are less likely to relapse if they receive a combination of medication, individual psychotherapy, and family therapy. In addition, people with bipolar illness are more likely to keep their illness under control if they receive family therapy.

Couples Therapy

Couples therapy tries to ease the tension your illness has created between you and your partner or spouse. Your partner is likely to take personally the symptoms of depression, such as lack of libido, withdrawal from other people, or loss of interest in life. If you have had mania or hypomania, your impulsive behavior may have hurt the other person. Couples therapy typically focuses on helping you and your partner discuss and solve such problems in a healthy way.

Improving your home life can help your individual treatment. Researchers have found that depressed women in happy marriages improve faster than women in unhappy marriages. Also, people with bipolar depression who receive couples therapy are less likely to relapse than those who do not receive therapy.

CHARTING YOUR ILLNESS

As part of your treatment, you and your doctor may create a chart to track the patterns of your illness. If your doctor decides to chart your illness, he or she will use lines on the chart to track your moods over many months. The line on your chart will curve up to show when you start to feel manic and down when you feel depressed. Over a year, your chart will be filled with a line that rises and falls in curves. At the same time, your doctor will track other aspects of your life: significant events, times you are hospitalized, how well you sleep, your energy levels, and the medication you take.

Understanding the patterns of your illness can help in many ways. Your chart may show that certain painful events trigger your illness, alerting you to discuss such events with your therapist. It may also reveal early signs of a new bout of illness that would otherwise go unnoticed. You may see that your sleep changed a few days before your mania returned. In the future, you will know that sleep changes mean you should call your doctor. Or you may learn that you tend to get sick in the fall and decide to take care to avoid stressful projects at that time of year. Over several years, your chart will reveal much about how often your illness recurs, the pattern your moods follow, the link between your moods and certain events, and the effectiveness of your medication or psychotherapy.

COMPLEMENTARY THERAPIES

Although doctors have made great strides in devising new medications for depressive illness, some people prefer to avoid drugs. You may be interested in trying to control your depression in ways that seem more natural. Complementary or alternative therapies for depression include herbal remedies, dietary supplements, relaxation techniques, and homeopathy.

Be aware that few well-designed scientific studies on alternative therapies have been performed. With few exceptions, most doctors consider alternative therapies unproven; that means they have not been proved to be effective through scientific studies.

If you are exploring or using alternative therapies, discuss your plans with your doctor. Tell your doctor if you plan to use an herbal remedy. He or she can advise you on whether it can be safely combined with other medication. In addition, your doctor may be able to suggest an effective dose, since herbal dosages and preparations are not standardized in the US and vary widely from brand to brand. Your doctor may recommend some lifestyle changes that complement conventional treatment, such as eating a healthy diet or getting regular exercise.

Herbal Remedies

A popular and well-known herbal remedy for depression is the plant *Hypericum perforatum,* commonly known as St John's wort. This herb is widely used to treat depression in Germany, where more than 2.7 million prescriptions for it were written in 1993. Some research suggests that when taken for mild or moderate depression, a standardized extract of St John's wort is as effective as antidepressants and has fewer side effects.

Researchers know very little about how St John's wort works or how safe it is for long-term use. Some research suggests that it acts similarly to an MAOI. There are drawbacks to use of this herb. St John's wort may interfere with how the body absorbs iron and other minerals. It may also cause heightened skin sensitivity to the sun, so use it with caution. St John's wort may take 4 to 6 weeks or longer to start working.

Several other herbs are believed to be useful for treating depression. *Ginkgo biloba* extract is thought to improve mood by boosting the amount of blood and oxygen your brain gets. Preparations of kava kava are used in Europe to treat anxiety, insomnia, and depression. Some people think drinking walnut tea can increase your brain's supply of serotonin, a neurotransmitter (chemical messenger) that helps regulate mood. Other herbs sometimes used for depression therapy are lemon balm, oat straw, and peppermint.

Diet and Dietary Supplements

Dietary supplements sometimes recommended to ease depression include the B vitamins, magnesium, zinc, folic acid, and the amino acid tyrosine. Discuss any supplement with your doctor before taking it, so that he or she can warn you of any dangers from a large dose of the supplement or from interactions with other medications. Tyrosine supplements, for example, can raise your blood pressure to dangerously high levels if you are also taking an MAOI antidepressant.

Dietary Recommendations

Some alternative practitioners recommend dietary changes to help depression. Eating complex carbohydrates may increase your brain's production of serotonin, the mood-regulating neurotransmitter. Complex carbohydrates include beans, bread, pasta, and whole grains.

Some practitioners think that a high-protein diet may boost your brain's supply of the neurotransmitters dopamine and norepinephrine, which also may improve your mood. Protein foods include meat, chicken, fish, beans, nuts, eggs, and tofu. Other practitioners, however, recommend a low-protein diet.

Other practitioners recommend eliminating sugar, caffeine, and alcohol; going easy on or eliminating fast foods and processed foods; and avoiding foods high in saturated fat.

Homeopathy

Homeopathy is an alternative medical system invented in the late 1700s by Samuel Hahnemann, a German physician and naturopath. Homeopathic remedies consist of specially prepared, extremely diluted doses of plant, animal, or mineral extracts. According to homeopathic theory, a dose of a substance that causes illness will, if sufficiently diluted, cure that illness by triggering the body's own healing energy or "vital force." The substance used may vary from person to person, depending on your symptoms, personality, and medical history. Homeopathic practitioners and some doctors claim that homeopathy can be effective for treating depression, though scant scientific evidence exists to support this assertion. Bach flower remedies, which also use homeopathic dilution, are popular among alternative practitioners for the treatment of mild mood disorders, including depression. Neither homeopathy nor Bach flower remedies have been proven effective by scientific research.

Other Alternative Therapies

Other nonstandard therapies and treatments for depression include deep breathing, massage therapy, and meditation. Some doctors recommend deep breathing to hold depression at bay. Deep breathing exercises increase the amount of oxygen that reaches your brain, which may lift your mood. Massage therapy has been used to treat depression triggered by painful events. Researchers have found that a 30-minute massage can lower levels of stress hormones, calm restlessness, and improve sleep.

Daily meditation may also help depression. When you meditate, you relax by focusing your mind on a particular item—your breath, a phrase or word repeated silently, an imaginary picture. According to one theory of psychology, depression comes from seeking too much stimulation. Meditation, according to this theory, helps you find emotional balance. Because it can take time for meditation to have an effect, this treatment requires a long-term commitment. Meditation probably has great value in helping to relieve stress, but it is unproven as a treatment for depression.

7

Helping a Loved One
With Depression

If your spouse, child, parent, or friend has depressive illness, you naturally want to help him or her get better. But no matter how long you have known the depressed person or how close you are to him or her, you may not know what is best to do about the problem. Should you talk about the illness or ignore it? What if something you say makes the depressed person feel worse? Is it a good idea to urge him or her to spend time with other people instead of being alone? If the depressed person is often irritable or angry, you may be in the habit of saying as little as possible. Maybe you wonder if it would be sensible to discuss your own worries with somebody who is already depressed. Despite your uncertainty, you can help a loved one through this time.

WHAT CAN I DO?

As a loving friend or family member of a person with depressive illness, you can do much to speed his or her recovery. It is important to realize, though, that you cannot get rid of your loved one's illness by talking to the person yourself. Depression needs professional medical care, just like any other illness.

The best thing you can do for someone with depression is to encourage him or her to seek out help. This is a simple matter if the ill person is your child; you simply call your family doctor and make an appointment. It can be much more difficult if the depressed person is a spouse, parent, or adult sibling who denies that anything is wrong. Once the illness has been diagnosed and treatment has begun, you can provide your loved one with non-judgmental emotional support and encouragement. It is also important to keep your family life and your own life balanced.

Encourage Your Loved One to Seek Help

If you want somebody you love to seek help, begin by telling him or her why you are worried. Describe the changes you have noticed in the person's mood, actions, and physical well-being. Ask questions that are open-ended rather than ones that can be answered with yes or no or a shake of the head. For example, instead of asking, "Are you depressed?" try "You seem so unhappy these days. What is going on?" If you are not convinced by the person's explanation, persist in urging him or her to seek help. You may have to bring up the topic several times before your loved one agrees.

If the depressed person is reluctant to see a doctor, offer to go along. Your offer demonstrates to the person that your concern is real. In addition, it turns the search for help into a team effort.

Plus, your observations could help the doctor to diagnose the illness accurately. Men are generally more reluctant to seek medical help for depression than women, though current wisdom holds that women get depressed more than men. If your partner refuses to see a doctor, try making an appointment anyway. Tell your partner the date and time well in advance and drive him or her to the doctor's office yourself. Your partner may not put up too much resistance, since depression tends to make people passive.

It may be difficult to be forceful if the depressed person is an older parent. Say, for example, that your mother seems to be depressed. If she is unaccustomed to taking advice from you, she may not be willing to listen to you. If she ignores or dismisses your concerns about her health, it may help if she hears the same message from several people. Try asking her close friends, her brothers and sisters, or her religious leader to talk to her. If this fails, try asking her doctor or a mental health specialist to phone her. If your mother accepts the call, the expert may be able to convince her that if she gets some help, she will soon feel better.

Once your loved one has been diagnosed with depression, your role in his or her treatment will vary. At a basic level, reassure the depressed person that he or she will get better. Remind your loved one that it takes time for treatment to have an effect. Second, you can help make sure the depressed person takes his or her medication correctly. If the doctor has prescribed several medications, you can help by sorting each day's pills into the correct combinations and doses. Try using plastic containers that have individual compartments for pills, available at most drugstores; these are especially useful for an older person. Third, watch for signs of improvement—you may be the first to notice. Mention any signs of improvement to your loved one as a means of reassuring him or her. If your loved one does not improve, suggest trying a new kind of treatment or seeking a second opinion.

Some doctors strongly believe in getting the depressed person's family involved in treatment. Family members can give doctors objective information about the depressed person's symptoms and medical history. Other doctors think that treatment for depression requires the same confidentiality that any other doctor–patient relationship does. In addition, the circumstances of the depression may decide your involvement. For example, say that your teenage daughter seems to be mildly depressed because she is struggling to separate from the family and become an independent adult. Unless her depression is more serious (for instance, if it included substance abuse problems or suicidal throughts), involving you in her treatment might make her feel worse. On the other hand, if it is your spouse or partner who has fallen ill, he or she may welcome your active involvement.

As your loved one enters treatment, learn as much as you can about his or her depressive illness. Look for other books on the subject and take advantage of the information offered by the organizations listed in the Resources section at the end of this book. Being well informed will aid you in helping your loved one.

Provide Emotional Support

Your emotional support—affection, understanding, patience, encouragement—combined with a gentle sense of humor can greatly help your loved one. Listen to what he or she says without judgment and do not try to talk the depression away.

If your loved one talks about feelings of failure and hopelessness, your immediate response may be to try to convince your loved one that he or she is not really depressed. You might think you should start by making a list of the person's blessings—a great job, a loving family, a nice house. But rather than lifting the person up, this pep talk may cast him or her down, adding to feelings of guilt, loneliness, and self-doubt. It is natural to try to cheer up someone who feels down but not necessarily helpful for a person with a depressive illness.

In a marriage or partnership, the partner should avoid saying or even thinking "You have me to love, so that's all you should need." Your partner's illness is not a personal criticism of you.

Avoid accusing the person of faking illness or engaging in self-pity or being selfish. Ordering the person "to snap out of it" is unlikely to be productive. Do not scoff or lecture. Instead, gently point out the reality of the situation without disparaging your loved one's feelings. Try to include him or her in fun activities, such as a walk on a nice day, a trip to the movies, or a visit to close friends.

However, avoid overwhelming the person with constant suggestions or pressure to join activities. Too many demands can make him or her feel anxious or increase his or her feelings of failure. This is a balancing act, and it takes practice. Say, for example, that your husband is going through a severe depression. Pushing him to attend your office party could make him more anxious. Yet leaving him alone for the evening may also make him feel worse.

Over time, you will learn to identify those times when your husband needs extra help or encouragement to extend himself and those when he does not. During periods of severe depression, he may rely on you in many ways. He may be unable to work, do chores around the house, or even get to the doctor's office without your help. You may quickly become used to treating him as helpless. But once he recovers, it is best to encourage him to assume as much responsibility as he can.

It may also be some time before you can confidently distinguish between your loved one's normal mood changes and those that result from illness. Some family members become overly vigilant, constantly looking for a mood that seems too high or low. This kind of vigilance can make your depressed loved one exceedingly anxious. It can also wear you out. It may become necessary to allow your loved one some privacy so that he or she will feel more at ease during recovery. Over time, as you learn about the illness and observe your loved one's moods, you will learn which signs are serious—any talk about suicide, for instance, is very serious—and which are not.

Take Care of Yourself and Your Family

Living with a depressed person can be difficult. Your loved one is likely to say hurtful things and demand much from you. A psychotherapist, counselor, or a support group made up of people and families who have been through similar experiences (see Chapter 5) can help you through this stressful time. Without such support, you have a chance of becoming depressed yourself.

Expect to feel angry or impatient with the depressed person sometimes. If the depressed person lives alone, ask other family members or friends to take turns checking in on him or her, so that the entire burden does not fall on you. If you take comfort in your own daily routine, try to maintain it.

When a person has depressive illness, it may be necessary to change the roles you play in your relationship with that person. Say, for example, that you have always been the breadwinner in the family and your spouse has always been the one who provides most of the emotional support to your children. But if your spouse becomes depressed, he or she will no longer be able to provide emotional support. As a result, you may have to become more involved in your children's emotional well-being as your spouse receives treatment. Such transitions typically take time for everyone involved.

In helping the depressed person, try not to forget about taking care of yourself. It is easy to let most of your attention and energy become focused on a loved one's depressive illness. If you feel that you are being forced to make too many sacrifices while you help your loved one, you may become irritable and eventually less tolerant. Make every effort to take care of the rest of your family, too. The extra attention that the depressed family member gets may foster tension in the household. Giving equal attention (as much as possible) to the activities of your healthy children can ease your own stress as well as theirs.

Doctors recommend discussing the depressive illness of a parent or a sibling with your children. Make the discussion as simple as needed for the child's age. Often, children take the illness personally. They may assume that they are responsible. They may think the depressed person is aloof because he or she no longer loves them. They need to understand that their loved one has an illness, that they did not cause it, and that it will get better.

In some cases, you may be able to help a depressed person with money or by allowing the person to move into your home. Some depressed people are disabled by their illness and can no longer support or care for themselves. This involves a commitment to help that the whole household needs to make.

WHEN A LOVED ONE IS HOSPITALIZED

Most of the time, your loved one will be treated as an outpatient in the office of a doctor or mental health specialist. Under certain conditions, however, your loved one may need treatment in a hospital. People who have threatened or attempted suicide are usually hospitalized. People with mania may also be hospitalized if their illness has brought on delusions or hallucinations or made them dangerously impulsive. Occasionally, the initial side effects of medication may be so severe that the depressed person needs hospital care. At other times, a doctor may wish to observe the depressed person as medication is started or withdrawn.

If your loved one needs to go to the hospital, he or she will probably do so voluntarily. However, say that your father, who is 68 years old, appears to have lost touch with reality, and is threatening to shoot someone with a pistol. People who appear to be in danger of harming themselves or others can be hospitalized against their wishes. Such hospitalization, known as involuntary care, is extremely upsetting. You will feel guilty if you send your father to the hospital involuntarily, especially if he is begging you not to. But you may be the only one standing between your father and the effects of his actions. Once he feels better, he may feel grateful. Laws governing involuntary care vary from state to state. For more information on involuntary care, call the depressed person's doctor, your state's attorney's office, the police, or the hospital emergency department.

It can be disturbing to visit your loved one in the hospital. At the hospital, you may see mentally ill people behaving in odd or unusual ways that may be symptoms of their illness.

It may be difficult dealing with your loved one. If he or she is deeply depressed, there may be long pauses after your questions. The person may be very angry about being put in the hospital. If your loved one is manic, it may be hard to understand what he or she is saying. Try dealing with your loved one honestly and firmly and explain the necessity of the treatment. Say that you brought the person to the hospital because he or she needed treatment.

In general, a person hospitalized for depressive illness will stay for only a short while. After he or she comes home, it may be a good idea to set out guidelines for the next bout of illness. If, for example, your partner has bipolar depression, he may agree that you should remove his credit cards or car keys the next time he gets sick. Discuss when and under what circumstances he would need to be hospitalized next. Draw up an agreement and get him to sign it. This will make things easier for you next time around. Some states allow more formal legal agreements, such as a durable power of attorney or another advance directive, to be drawn up in these instances, but that requires an attorney.

WHEN A LOVED ONE IS SUICIDAL

Myths About Suicide

Suicidal thoughts can be a symptom of moderate to severe depressive illness, though most people who are depressed do not kill themselves. Depressive illness is one of the leading risk factors for attempted suicide. Almost all people who kill themselves have a mental illness or a substance abuse problem; most have more than one. Other risk factors, described below, are often also present.

A common misconception about suicide is that people who talk about it do not attempt it. If your loved one talks about suicide, he or she is asking for help and may be serious about his or her intentions. Any talk of suicide must be taken very seriously.

Do not assume that suicide cannot occur in your family. People of all ages and all social and economic groups attempt suicide. You can do yourself and your loved one with a depressive illness a favor by learning the warning signs of suicide.

Clues and Risk Factors

A number of different factors can affect a person's risk of suicide. Certain clues can tell you when a depressed family member or friend is thinking of suicide. For example, a detailed suicide plan, a threat of suicide, talk of death or despair, or a preoccupation with death indicate suicidal thoughts. A loved one who withdraws from family and friends, who abuses drugs or alcohol, or whose behavior suddenly becomes violent may be suicidal. Giving away valued possessions or making final arrangements, such as completing a will, can be a sign. A person whose behavior changes abruptly—who suddenly seems happy after months of depression or is suddenly galvanized after prolonged apathy—may have decided to kill himself or herself. In children, running away from home or a sudden change in school performance can point to suicidal thoughts. Many of the symptoms of depression—anxiety, tension, withdrawal from others, inability to concentrate, feeling worthless, physical complaints, sleep changes, changes in appetite—are also seen in people who kill themselves.

- **Marital status.** A person's marital status also affects the likelihood of suicide. People who are single, widowed, separated, or divorced are at greater risk for suicide than are married people.
- **Age and sex.** A person's age and sex also factor into his or her risk for suicide. The risk of suicide generally increases with age. An estimated 60 percent of all people who commit suicide are over age 60, and most of them are men. Suicide is also notably higher in young people between the ages of 15 and 24. More men than women die by suicide (4.5 men to 1 woman in 1994), though women are more likely than men to attempt suicide unsuccessfully (about 2 women to every man in 1994). One explanation may be that men generally choose more lethal means, such as guns, whereas women tend to try less lethal means, such as pills.
- **Health status.** A person's health can make him or her more likely to commit suicide. People who have recently had major surgery, who are in great pain, or who have a long-lasting or terminal illness are at high risk. As already mentioned, mental illness and substance abuse problems are important risk factors.
- **Family dysfunction.** Sexual or physical abuse that occurred within the family is a risk factor, as is a history of other family members who have or have had mental illnesses or substance abuse problems or who have committed suicide.
- **Prior suicide attempts.** Those who have attempted suicide before are at risk for doing so again.
- **Suicides of others.** Knowledge of or exposure to the suicide deaths of others, whether family members or people read about in books or news media, can be a risk factor. Adolescents may be at risk when friends or schoolmates kill themselves. (Some depressed people may be "inspired" to follow through on their thoughts by reading news accounts of other suicides.)

APPROACHING YOUR LOVED ONE

The best way to know if your loved one is thinking of suicide is to ask. Do not worry about planting the idea of suicide in his or her mind. Talking about suicide does *not* encourage it. Rather, giving the person an opportunity to talk through strong fears and negative emotions can help him or her feel less alone. Talking can actually decrease your loved one's risk. Ask direct, caring questions: Have you thought about dying? Do you ever think about hurting yourself? How would you do it? When would you do it? Where would you do it? You may find that the depressed person would like to be dead but has not thought further than that. Or you may find that your loved one already has a detailed plan. Either way, contact the person's doctor, bring the person to an emergency department, or call 911 or your emergency medical services number.

Try not to blame the depressed person for these feelings. Remind your loved one that these thoughts are a part of his or her illness. Let the person know his or her life is important. At the same time, take precautions and eliminate any dangerous objects from the environment. Lock up or dispose of guns, medication (both prescription and over-the-counter), alcohol, knives, and anything else he or she can use.

If you suspect that your loved one has suicidal feelings but refuses to talk about them, contact the person's doctor or a mental health specialist for advice. Try to persuade your loved one to see a psychiatrist or other mental health specialist.

Sometimes talk of suicide and suicide attempts occur after treatment has begun. Severely depressed people who may not have had the energy to commit suicide may find that they have enough energy to carry out their impulses shortly after their treatment begins taking effect. Do not assume that your loved one will not commit suicide because he or she seems to be getting better.

WHEN A CHILD IS DEPRESSED

Until the 1960s, doctors thought it was impossible for children or adolescents to develop depressive illness. Today, we know that this theory is wrong. Some research studies suggest that between 3 million and 6 million Americans under the age of 18 have depressive illness. Untreated depression is just as serious in young people as it is in an older person. Almost 2,000 people between the ages of 15 and 19 are known to have killed themselves in 1993, although experts think the true number may be much higher because suicide is widely underreported. And for every young person who commits suicide, at least 8 others attempt it.

Children of any age can have depressive illness, but having it becomes more likely as they get older. Some experts think even babies can get depressed if they are abused, neglected, or separated from their mothers. Babies who fail to develop at the normal rate may actually be depressed. Researchers have found that among children aged 12 and younger, between 1 percent and 2 percent are depressed. This percentage jumps during adolescence, when it is thought about 8 percent of boys and 10 percent of girls become depressed. The rate of depression among girls climbs steeply during their teen years, so that by the end of adolescence about twice as many girls as boys are depressed. In addition, bipolar illness often strikes for the first time during a person's teens, frequently first as depression rather than mania.

Many researchers think that depressive illnesses among children are widely unnoticed and untreated. Picking up a child's depression can be difficult even for the most caring and sensitive parents. A certain amount of sadness, turmoil, and social withdrawal is normal at different stages of childhood. And while depressed children usually have the same symptoms as depressed adults, they do not always show them in the same way. Many depressed children complain of physical ailments, such as headaches or stomachaches, rather than feelings of sadness. Others talk about feeling stupid, ugly, or useless. Still others reveal their depression through behavior problems, such as fighting, having trouble at school, bed-wetting, or abusing substances.

Bipolar depression, including mania, sometimes begins in childhood. The symptoms of mania most commonly seen in children are hyperactivity, distractibility, rushed speech, trouble sleeping, being easily frustrated, and indulging in outbursts of rage. Mania in young people is often misdiagnosed as attention-deficit hyperactivity disorder (ADHD), a condition also marked by hyperactivity and impulsive behavior.

If you think your child is depressed, you may have to watch him or her carefully for several weeks to make sure his or her mood is outside what is considered normal. It may help to ask the child's teacher for his or her impression. If you continue to feel worried, make an appointment with your child's doctor. If he or she cannot find a physical cause for the depression, ask for a referral to a mental health specialist. Ideally, a depressed child should be treated by a professional who specializes in treating children.

Spotting depressive illness can be more difficult in adolescents. Bipolar depression often emerges at this time in life, yet its symptoms—impulsive behavior, irritability, loss of control—can seem normal in teenagers. One clue to depression is persistent signs of change or withdrawal. If your teen used to be outgoing but is now always alone, he or she may have a depressive illness. The good student who begins failing and the normally cheerful teen who is now routinely irritable could also be depressed. If you are worried about your adolescent and he or she seems unwilling to talk with you, it may be a good idea to talk to his or her best friend. Your talk may not yield satisfying results, since teenagers often close ranks against adults. However, your child's friend may know about any suicidal feelings your child has and may be willing to share his or her concerns with you.

Your adolescent may be unwilling to see a doctor, in which case it will be up to you to insist that he or she find help. Early treatment can avoid years of unnecessary suffering.

If your child is clinically depressed, the treatment your doctor recommends may vary with the child's age. Psychotherapy is usually the first choice, in particular cognitive therapy (see Chapter 6). Counselors who are trained to speak on a child's level will try to discover what is disturbing the child and will help find solutions. Often, this therapy involves parents because they can help make the changes required to help the child.

If your adolescent is showing signs of bipolar illness, he or she may be treated with such medication as lithium. A teenager with major depression may be prescribed antidepressants. In younger children, the use of antidepressants is much less well studied. Few antidepressants have been developed or tested with children in mind, although a recent study of 96 children found that fluoxetine (Prozac) was as effective a treatment for major depression in children as it is in adults. Young people's bodies may metabolize (process) these drugs in a different way than do adults' bodies, and they may be more prone to side effects. Therefore, careful medical supervision—including monitoring of the dose—is crucial.

Acknowledging that your child has depressive illness is guilt-provoking and heart-wrenching. It is useful to remember, however, that by getting your child help right away, you could be sparing him or her years of future suffering.

WHEN AN OLDER PERSON IS DEPRESSED

Depressive illness is widespread among older people. According to one large study, about 15 percent of people over age 65 have some symptoms of depression. Mania can also emerge in older people, although it is uncommon. Despite the prevalence of depression among older people, their illness typically goes untreated. By one estimate, only about 10 percent of older people who need psychiatric treatment ever receive it. This may stem from the fact that many people, including some doctors, mistake symptoms of depression as a normal part of aging. But just as with younger people, depression among older people is an illness that can be healed with treatment.

No one knows exactly how many older Americans are depressed because estimates vary widely. But researchers have concluded that depression tends to affect people in nursing homes more than it does people who live at home. An estimated 3 percent of older people living at home have major depression, whereas 15 percent to 25 percent of older people in nursing homes have major or minor depression. This rate of depression has led to a high rate of suicide among older people, especially among white men.

One reason depressive illness often goes untreated in older people is because many older people consider their depression normal. They have, after all, contended with many losses—the end of their careers, the death of good friends or a beloved mate, the ebbing of good health. Depression may seem like a reasonable response to these losses. In addition, depression shows itself differently in older people than in younger adults. Older depressed people are less likely to complain of sadness and more likely to mention aches and pain, constipation, or fatigue. Many older people have physical health problems that may get more of their attention than the depression does. Finally, depressed older people are likely to be misdiagnosed as having dementia.

There are several ways you can help your loved one get treatment for depression. If your loved one is depressed, he or she will first need a complete physical checkup. You can help by urging him or her to get a checkup. If the older person is withdrawn or confused, go with him or her to the doctor's office and provide information about the person's medical history. The doctor will check whether a physical illness is causing the depression and will ask about all the drugs, both prescription and nonprescription, that the older person uses. Many of these drugs can cause depression, either by themselves or by reacting with each other. If the doctor finds no physical reason why the older person is depressed, your loved one should probably see a mental health specialist. Ideally, you should find someone who specializes in the mental health of older people or at least has experience in treating older people. If you think your loved one may have both dementia and depression, it is helpful for him or her to see a geriatric psychiatrist—an MD who can diagnose and treat all types of illness in older people.

To treat depressive illness in older people, many doctors recommend a combination of medication and short-term psychotherapy. Prescribing antidepressants for an older person can be tricky because older people's bodies may metabolize medications in a different way than do younger people's bodies. Generally, older people end up retaining much more of the drug in their system. This means that older people can overdose on an amount that would not bother a younger person. In addition, they are more likely to suffer side effects. Another drawback is that antidepressants can aggravate other medical conditions, such as heart disease. As a result, the older person with depression and his or her doctor should choose an antidepressant carefully.

RECOVERY

Depressive illness is not easy for anyone, whether you have the illness or care about someone who does. The illness changes a person's thoughts, actions, physical health, and emotions, causing disruption in the lives of their spouses, partners, relatives, and friends. But almost everyone can recover from depressive illness. For some people, the illness may go and never return. Others may need to make a lifelong effort of controlling it with medication, psychotherapy, education, good physical care, or any combination of therapies. Either way, recovery is on the horizon.

Resources

The organizations listed below can provide useful information, products, and services for people who have depression.

Agency for Health Care Policy and Research (AHCPR)
AHCPR Publications Clearinghouse
P.O. Box 8547
Silver Spring, MD 20907-8547
phone: (800) 358-9295

E-MAIL:
  info@ahcpr.gov

WEB SITE:
  http://www.ahcpr.gov/

> The AHCPR is a government agency charged with supporting research designed to improve the quality of health care, reduce its cost, and broaden access to essential services. The agency has developed a number of clinical practice guidelines, including one on the treatment of depression. Versions for both professionals and consumers are available online and in print.

American Academy of Child and Adolescent Psychiatry
3615 Wisconsin Avenue, NW
Washington, DC 20016-3007
phone: (800) 333-7636

WEB SITE:
  http://www.aacap.org

> This professional association provides free information and referrals to psychiatrists specializing in children and adolescents.

American Association of Suicidology
4201 Connecticut Avenue, NW, suite 310
Washington, DC 20008
phone: (202) 237-2280

E-MAIL:
 amyj@tx.netcom.com

WEB SITE:
 http://www.cyberpsych.org

> This nonprofit organization provides free information and referrals to crisis centers and support groups.

American Psychiatric Association
1400 K Street, NW
Washington, DC 20005
phone: (202) 682-6220

WEB SITE:
 http://www.psych.org

> This professional association provides free information on mental disorder issues and referrals to state psychiatric societies, which can make referrals to local practitioners.

American Psychological Association
750 First Street, NE
Washington, DC 20002-4242
phone: (202) 336-5500

WEB SITE:
 http://www.apa.org

> This professional association provides free material on mental disorders and referrals.

AMI Québec
5253 boul. Décarie
bureau 150
Montréal, Quebec
H3W 3C3
phone: (514) 486-1448

AMI Québec is a grass-roots support and advocacy organization for families and friends of people with mental illnesses. Located in Montréal, it offers a variety of self-help groups, seminars, education programs, and other resources, primarily for the English-speaking population.

Canadian Medical Association
1867 Alta Vista Drive
Ottawa, ON
K1G 3Y6
phone: (613) 731-9331

WEB SITE:
http://www.cma.ca

The Canadian Medical Association is a valuable source of medical information and resources, geared mainly toward the professional. The group's web site contains a search engine that will help you locate links to specific medical topics, including depression.

Center for Cognitive Therapy
3600 Market Street, 8th floor
Philadelphia, PA 19104-2649
phone: (215) 898-4100

WEB SITE:
http://www.med.upen.edu/psycct

This organization, which is part of the University of Pennsylvania, provides referrals to cognitive therapists worldwide.

Clarke Institute of Psychiatry
Division of the Addiction and Mental Health Services Corporation
250 College Street
Toronto, Ontario
Canada M5T 1R8
phone: (416) 979-2221

WEB SITE:
http://www.clarke-inst.on.ca./home.html

The Clarke Institute of Psychiatry, affiliated with the University of Toronto, is a research center for mental health issues. The center offers treatment programs, continuing education seminars, and free informational literature.

Depression and Related Affective Disorders Association (DRADA)
Meyer 3-181, 600 N. Wolfe Street
Baltimore, MD 21287-7381
phone: (410) 955-4647 (Baltimore)
(202) 995-5800 (Washington, DC)

E-MAIL:
drada-g@welchlink.welch.jhv.edu

WEB SITE:
http://www.med.jhv.edu/drada

This nonprofit organization provides free information on mood disorders and sponsors workshops and support groups, mainly in the Baltimore–District of Columbia area.

Depression/Awareness, Recognition, and Treatment (D/ART)
5600 Fishers Lane
Rockville, MD 20857
phone: (800) 421-4211

WEB SITE:
http://www.nimh.nih.gov/dart/

This program, sponsored by the National Institute of Mental Health, provides an educational program on depressive illnesses for the public and professionals.

Federation of Families for Children's Mental Health
1021 Prince Street
Alexandria, VA 22314-2971
phone: (703) 684-7710

E-MAIL:
ffcmh@crosslink.net

WEB SITE:

http://www.ffcmh.org

This national parent-run, nonprofit organization focuses on the needs of children and youth with emotional, behavioral, or mental disorders and provides free information to their families.

Health Canada
A.L. 0913A
Ottawa, Canada
K1A 0K9
phone: (613) 941-5336

WEB SITE:

http://www.hc-sc.gc.ca

Health Canada is the federal department responsible for helping Canadians maintain their health. The department promotes disease prevention and healthy living. You can search Health Canada's medical database for information on specific health-related topics, including depression.

National Alliance for the Mentally Ill
200 N. Glebe Road, suite 1015
Arlington, VA 22203-3754
phone: (800) 950-6264
TDD: (703) 516-7991

WEB SITE:

http://www.nami.org

This nonprofit association is the umbrella organization for more than 1,000 local support and advocacy groups for families and individuals affected by serious mental disorders. It provides support to families and free information on mental disorders.

National Depressive and Manic Depressive Association
730 N. Franklin, suite 501
Chicago, IL 60610-3526
phone: (800) 826-3632

E-MAIL:
myrtis@aol.com

WEB SITE:
http://www.ndmda.org

This nonprofit organization provides referrals to support groups and free information on depression and manic depressive illness.

National Foundation for Depressive Illness
P.O. Box 2257
New York, NY 10116
phone: (800) 248-4344 or (800) 239-1265

WEB SITE:
http://www.depression.org

This nonprofit organization supplies recorded information on the symptoms of depressive illness and how to get help; it also provides referrals.

National Institute of Mental Health
Public Inquiries Office
5600 Fishers Lane, room 7C-02, MSC 8030
Bethesda, MD 20892-8030
phone: (301) 443-4513; for free brochures, (800) 421-4211

E-MAIL:
nimhinfo@nih.gov

WEB SITE:
http://www.nimh.nih.gov/

This federal research organization provides free information on depression and other mental disorders through a number of programs, including Depression/Awareness, Recognition, and Treatment (D/ART, listed on page 212) and its web site.

National Mental Health Association
1021 Prince Street
Alexandria, VA 22314-2971
phone: (800) 969-6642

WEB SITE:

http://www.nmha.org

This nonprofit organization provides information on mental health topics, referrals to mental health providers, a directory of national network of local mental health associations, and more.

National Mental Health Services Knowledge Exchange Network (KEN)
P.O. Box 42490
Washington, DC 20015
phone: (800) 789-2647
TDD: (301) 443-9006

E-MAIL:

ken@mentalhealth.org

WEB SITE:

http://www.mentalhealth.org

This agency—which is run by the Center for Mental Health Services, part of the US Department of Health and Human Services (USDHHS)—provides the *Mental Health Directory,* a state-by-state listing of mental health facilities, and other free information.

National Organization for SAD (NOSAD)
P.O. Box 451
Vienna, VA 22180

This nonprofit organization provides free information on seasonal affective disorder (SAD).

Glossary

This glossary defines terms that your doctor may have mentioned or that you may have come across while reading about depression. Italicized words within entries refer you to other entries for more information.

A

akathisia: Restlessness, a side effect of *antipsychotic drugs*.

akinesia: Stiff movements, a side effect of *antipsychotic drugs*.

amygdala: Part of the brain's *limbic system* that interprets emotions and controls responses to emotions.

anhedonia: Loss or lack of interest in pleasurable activities, a symptom of *depressive illness*.

antianxiety drugs: Medication, also called sedative or hypnotic drugs, sometimes used to treat symptoms of *depressive illness*.

anticholinergic effects: A group of side effects caused by *tricyclic antidepressant drugs* that include dry mouth, constipation, difficulty urinating, problems with vision, and a racing heart.

anticonvulsant drugs: Originally developed to treat seizures, these drugs also help control *bipolar depression*.

antidepressant drugs: These medications alleviate *depressive illness*.

antipsychotic drugs: Used to treat people who have lost touch with reality during *depressive illness*; also called *neuroleptic drugs*.

atypical depression: A form of *depressive illness* with a mix of symptoms, some typical of *major depression* (sadness) and some not typical (overeating and oversleeping).

axon: Part of a brain's nerve cell, or *neuron,* that forwards messages to another *neuron.*

B

behavior therapy: A form of *psychotherapy* based on the idea that *depressive illness* is a kind of behavior that is learned and can be unlearned.

biogenic amines: *Neurotransmitters,* namely *norepinephrine,* serotonin, and dopamine, suspected of playing a role in causing *depressive illness.*

biological clock: A mechanism that controls natural rhythms in the body, such as a regular rise and fall in body temperature.

bipolar depression: Also known as manic depression, manic-depressive illness, and bipolar disorder; this is a form of *depressive illness* in which *depression* alternates with *mania* (euphoria).

bipolar I: A form of *bipolar depression* in which moods swing between the extremes of *depression* and *mania.*

bipolar II: A form of *bipolar depression* in which moods swing between *depression* and *hypomania* (mild *mania*).

C

cell body: Part of the brain's nerve cells, or *neurons.*

chromosomes: Threadlike structures in the center of a body cell that contain *genes.*

circadian rhythms: Natural biological cycles that occur in the human body about once every 24 hours; see *biological clock.*

clang association: Choosing words for their sounds rather than their meanings; sometimes a symptom of *mania.*

clinical depression: See *major depression.*

coexisting depression: *Depression* that occurs in the presence of another illness.

cognitive therapy: A short-term *psychotherapy* based on the assumption that negative thinking largely causes *depressive illness.*

couples therapy: A form of *psychotherapy* that aims to ease tension between the depressed person and his or her partner or spouse.

cyclothymia: A milder form of *bipolar depression* in which moods swing between *hypomania* and mild *depression;* also called cyclothymic disorder.

D

delusion: Firm belief in something contradicted by fact.

dendrites: Part of the brain's *neurons;* branching fibers that pick up messages.

denial: The inability to acknowledge an illness, which is itself a symptom of that illness.

depression: Another word for *depressive illness,* although many people use the word *depression* to describe everyday feelings of sadness.

depressive illness: A *mood disorder* marked primarily by extreme sadness, also known as *depression.* Other symptoms can include lack of interest in everyday or pleasurable activities; distorted thoughts of low-self esteem, worthlessness, or hopelessness; fatigue; insomnia; loss of appetite; and possibly thoughts of suicide. *Bipolar depression* is a depressive illness.

dexamethasone suppression test (DST): A test of how the body handles a dose of a dexamethasone, a synthetic version of the hormone cortisol. About half of all people with *depression* have an abnormal response to the dose; thus, the test is used to help confirm rather than determine a diagnosis.

diurnal variation of mood: A tendency for depressed people to feel worse at a particular time of day, usually first thing in the morning.

DNA (deoxyribonucleic acid): A complex protein found in *chromosomes* that carries genetic information.

dysphoria: Also called dysphoric mood, the bleak sad mood of *depressive illness*.

dysphoric mania: A subdued or unhappy form of *mania*.

dysthymia: A chronic (long-lasting) but less intense form of *depressive illness*.

dystonic reaction: Muscle contractions that cause involuntary movements of the face, neck, tongue, back, and eyes; a side effect of *antipsychotic drugs*.

E

electroconvulsive therapy (ECT): Also known as shock treatment, ECT is an effective and fast-acting treatment for *depressive illness* and *mania*. ECT works by sending a low electrical signal through the brain, inducing a general seizure when a person is under general anesthesia.

electroencephalograph (EEG): An instrument used to study sleep by measuring and recording the electrical waves emitted by the brain.

endocrine system: The body's system of *hormone*-producing *glands*.

episode: A discrete period of *depressive illness* or *mania*.

F

family therapy: A form of *psychotherapy* that educates family members about *depressive illness*, examines their feelings toward the depressed person, and shows how they can help in treatment.

family-care doctor: A doctor who diagnoses and treats most health problems for people of all ages.

G

gene mapping: A process in which scientists try to locate a particular *gene* for a trait on a particular *chromosome*.

gene markers: Particular variations on *chromosomes.* Because they are inherited along with a specific *gene,* they may mark the location of that *gene* on the *chromosome.*

genes: Individual units of genetic information contained on *chromosomes.* Genes influence and direct the development of specific physical or biochemical characteristics.

glands: Body organs that produce chemicals for the body's use, including enzymes and *hormones.*

H

hallucination: Seeing, hearing, tasting, touching, or smelling something that is not actually there.

hippocampus: Part of the brain's *limbic system* that interprets emotions and responses to emotions.

homeopathy: An alternative medical system, originating in the 1700s, in which specially prepared, extremely diluted doses of plant, animal, or mineral extracts are given to trigger the body's own healing energy or "vital force."

hormones: Substances secreted by *glands* that control such physical processes as growth and sexual development.

hypermania: An intense form of mania, sometimes a symptom of *bipolar depression.*

hypersexuality: Increased sexuality, often a symptom of *bipolar depression.*

hypersomnia: Increased need for sleep, sometimes a symptom of *depressive illness.*

hypomania: A mild form of *mania,* sometimes a symptom of *bipolar depression.*

hypothalamus: A part of the brain that controls appetite, sleep, sexual desire, body temperature, reactions to stress, the timing of many other functions, and the *pituitary gland.*

I

insomnia: Sleeplessness, often a symptom of *depressive illness.*

interpersonal therapy: A form of *psychotherapy* that focuses on solving problems in relationships that may cause or prolong *depressive illness.*

L

labile affect: Sudden changes in mood or behavior, often a symptom of *mania.*

light therapy: Sometimes called phototherapy, light therapy treats *seasonal affective disorder (SAD)* with bright lights designed to compensate for the loss of daylight in winter.

limbic system: A particular brain area that regulates emotions, physical drives (such as sexuality), and response to stress.

lymphocytes: Substances in the blood, produced by lymph *glands,* that protect the body against disease.

M

major affective disorders: A group of illnesses that affect mood, including *depressive illness;* also called *mood disorders.*

major depression: The most common form of *depressive illness,* marked by prolonged sadness, loss of pleasure, or both, and additional changes in emotion, thought, behavior, and physical well-being.

mania: A *mood disorder* characterized by overactivity, irritability, or euphoria; a symptom or stage of *bipolar depression.*

masked depression: *Depressive illness* that appears as some other disorder, such as substance abuse or chronic aches and pains.

melancholia: Another term for the overwhelming sadness and grief of *depressive illness.*

melatonin: Hormone secreted during the night by a part of the brain called the pineal gland. Stimulated by darkness and suppressed by light, melatonin is believed to contribute to *seasonal affective disorder (SAD)*.

mental disorder: A general term used to describe an illness of the mind or emotions, including *depression*. *Mood disorders* are one category of mental disorder; among several other categories are anxiety disorders, such as panic attacks; psychotic disorders, such as schizophrenia; and eating disorders, such as bulimia.

metabolites: Substances left over after the body has used certain *neurotransmitters* found in the blood, urine, and other body fluids.

minor depression: Also called minor depressive disorder, this is an illness similar to *major depression* but with milder symptoms.

mixed state: A form of *bipolar depression* in which people experience *depression* and mania at the same time.

monoamine oxidase inhibitors (MAOIs): *Antidepressant drugs* that work by preventing the breakdown of certain *neurotransmitters* in the brain.

mood congruent: Referring to *hallucinations* or *delusions;* having a tone or content that is in keeping with the person's mood.

mood disorders: Also known as affective disorders, a group of illnesses that disrupt normal moods. *Depressive illness* is a mood disorder.

mood incongruent: Referring to *hallucinations* or *delusions;* having a tone or content that is not in keeping with the person's mood.

mood stabilizers: Drugs used to subdue *mania* and lift *depressive illness.* Lithium is a mood stabilizer.

N

nerve impulses: The form in which messages travel throughout the brain, from one *neuron* to another.

neuroleptic drugs: See *antipsychotic drugs.*

neurons: Nerve cells in the brain and spinal cord.

neurotransmitters: Chemicals used to carry messages throughout the brain's network of cells.

non-REM sleep: Non–rapid eye movement sleep; the phase of sleep in which mental activity slows but does not stop. During this phase, the brain emits slower but larger and larger brain waves.

noncompliance: Failure to take medication as prescribed.

norepinephrine: A *neurotransmitter* (chemical messenger) in the brain, believed to help regulate moods.

nurse practitioner: A professional nurse with additional training who performs tasks formerly reserved for doctors.

O

orthostatic hypotension: Feeling lightheaded or dizzy after standing up quickly, a feeling due to blood's pooling in the lower extremities and causing temporary low blood pressure; a side effect of *tricyclic antidepressant drugs*.

P

physician assistant: Someone with medical knowledge who is not a doctor but works under a doctor's supervision.

pituitary gland: The body's master *gland* that controls many important *hormones*.

postpartum depression: A form of *depressive illness*—with the same symptoms as *major depression*—that develops in approximately 10 percent of new mothers about 1 week to 6 months after they give birth to their babies.

postpartum psychosis: A severe form of *postpartum depression* that occurs in 1 or 2 of every 1,000 new mothers. Its symptoms include *hallucinations*, *delusions*, and suicidal thoughts.

premenstrual dysphoric disorder: A cyclic illness that affects some 3 percent to 5 percent of menstruating women. Women with this illness feel deeply depressed and irritable for 1 or 2 weeks before menstruation each month.

pressure of speech: Rapid and confusing speech, a symptom of *mania*.

psychiatric disorder: A medical condition that affects the mind; also called *mental disorder*.

psychiatric nurse: A professional nurse who specializes in treating *mental disorders*.

psychiatrist: A physician who specializes in diagnosing and treating *mental disorders*. Only physicians can prescribe medication.

psychoanalysis: An intensive, usually long-lasting kind of *psychotherapy* that tries to change a person's personality rather than simply alleviate symptoms.

psychologist: An expert in the mind and how it works. Psychologists do not prescribe medication.

psychomotor agitation: Speeding up of movements, sometimes a symptom of *depressive illness*.

psychomotor retardation: Slowing of speech and movements, often a symptom of *depressive illness*.

psychotherapy: A common treatment for *depressive illness*, either by itself or in combination with medication, in which the depressed person and a therapist talk through emotions, problems, and life experiences in an attempt to treat the symptoms of *depression*.

psychotic depression: *Depressive illness* with *delusions* or *hallucinations*; develops in about 15 percent of people with *major depression*.

R

rapid cycling: A form of *bipolar depression* in which people suffer four or more episodes in 1 year.

receptor: A kind of landing dock on the surface of a nerve cell in the brain where a *neurotransmitter* fits after carrying a message from another nerve cell.

recurrence: The beginning of a new episode of *depressive illness.*

recurrent brief depressive disorder: A form of *depressive illness* in which the symptoms are as severe as in *major depression* but last for only a brief time.

relapse: The return of *depressive illness* after treatment begins.

REM sleep: Rapid eye movement sleep, the phase of sleep in which dreams occur. During this phase, the sleeping person's eyes move rapidly, heartbeat and breathing become irregular, and brain waves become small and fast, similar to those of an awake person.

reuptake: The process by which a *neuron* reabsorbs a *neurotransmitter* after it has done its job.

S

seasonal affective disorder (SAD): A type of *depressive illness* that occurs only at certain times of the year. People with SAD usually feel lethargic and depressed during the winter and normal or unusually happy during the summer.

sedation: Used in referring to the side effects of *antidepressant drugs*—sleepiness or drowsiness.

selective serotonin reuptake inhibitors (SSRIs): *Antidepressant drugs* that work by preventing the reuptake of the *neurotransmitter* serotonin.

self-medication: The process of abusing alcohol or drugs in order to relieve symptoms.

shortened REM latency: Abnormal sleep, in which the REM (rapid eye movement, or dream) phase occurs much earlier in the night than usual; often found in depressed people.

social worker: A person trained to help you solve problems.

somatic symptoms: The symptoms of *depressive illness* that affect the body, such as sleep changes.

subsyndromal depression: A milder form of *depressive illness* with fewer than five symptoms.

summer depression: A form of *depressive illness* in which people lose their appetites, have trouble sleeping, and feel anxious and agitated during the summer. In winter, they feel normal or unusually happy.

synapse: A gap that lies between one *neuron* and the next in the brain.

syndrome: An illness characterized by a collection of symptoms that occur together.

T

tardive dyskinesia: Involuntary movements of the mouth, head, and body; a serious side effect of long-term use of *antipsychotic drugs*.

terminal insomnia: Waking extremely early in the morning, often a symptom of depression.

thyroid-releasing hormone (TRH) stimulation test: A test showing whether the system by which the thyroid secretes thyroid hormone is working normally. This process is abnormal in about 30 percent to 60 percent of severely depressed people; thus, this test is used to confirm rather than determine a diagnosis of *depression*.

trazodone: A newer *antidepressant drug,* sometimes called an atypical antidepressant because it is chemically different from older antidepressants.

tricyclic antidepressant (TCA) drugs: Medications that improve moods by blocking the *reuptake* of certain *neurotransmitters*.

U

unipolar depression: Another term for *major depression,* used to distinguish it from *bipolar depression*.

V

vegetative symptoms: The physical symptoms of *depressive illness,* such as restlessness and psychomotor retardation.

Index

Please note: Medications are indexed by generic name only.